30 Day Whole Food Challenge

Complete Guide of 30 Day Whole Food Diet for Beginners to Have a Healthy Lifestyle

Barbara Amanda

Table of Contents

Introduction

I wish to personally thank you and congratulate you for reading the book, "30 Day Whole Food Challenge".

If you spend lots of time on health blogs, health magazines, or social media, you've probably heard of the Whole30. You might have seen some of the incredible before and after weight loss images or know something about the awesome health benefits that comes with the diet. From fighting sugar addiction to discovering food sensitivities, it seems there's nothing the Whole30 cannot do. This is the only book you will need to unlock the secrets of the Whole30 and finally become healthy!

So, exactly what is the Whole30 diet? Well, the Whole30 is a diet where for 30 days you stop consuming specific food groups. The goal of the Whole30 is to renew your health, eating habits, and relationship with food. The Whole30 is created to assist you to reevaluate how you eat and better understand how various foods make you feel. But it is an incredibly restrictive diet, so it is not a long-term lifestyle plan.

This book will allow you to make some of the tastiest healthy meals on the planet and more. The book features all sorts of recipes and instructions for preparing them. The nutritional information is also given for each recipe. We have done our very best to include a diverse set of recipes to satisfy your taste buds each day. Here you will find meals ready to be served for breakfast, lunches, dinners. These recipes specialize in chicken, meat, beef, pork, fish and seafood, soups and stews, vegan and vegetarian, appetizers and side dishes, and desserts for the Whole30.

In chapter 2 of this book, you will find the 30 days Whole Food meal plan, which will help make the road for your health goals much easier. Use this book daily as it contains a diverse set of healthy and delicious recipes that will satisfy your stomach, make you feel better and lose weight!

Thank you again for purchasing and reading this book, I hope that you will enjoy it!

How the Whole30 Changed My Life

Back in March 2016, I didn't realize that my life was about to dramatically change for the better. I used to be a binge eater. I was overweight and ate junk food whenever I can. This made me emotionally unstable and crippled my self-esteem. I wanted to change my life but I was clueless about diets and exercise and how to start becoming healthy. I later attempted on various diets such as the Paleo diet, Ketogenic diet, and Weight Watchers, but it just wasn't right for me.

One day while surfing the Internet I stumbled across an article about the Whole30. I was curious and begin researching more about the program. My main goal was to lose weight, and while I know the Whole30 diet wasn't designed solely for that purpose I figured I had nothing to lose. I was sick of being miserable, sick of all this negative thinking, sick of feeling disgusted at myself, and sick of being addicted to sugar. I made a commitment to stick to the Whole30 program to the bitter end.

I started the Whole30 in November and followed the diet strictly for the entire month. I stopped drinking coffee, only drank water, ate only eggs for breakfast, and prepared a delicious dinner using my Instant Pot each day. I was genuinely excited about eating vegetables and fruit. I was also looking forward preparing all my meals from home.

What happened to me after the Whole30 include:

- I lost around 40 pounds. Side note: I didn't actually record my weight before beginning the Whole30, but going off my last recorded weight, I'm 40 pounds lighter. Without a doubt, I lost more weight on the Whole30 than the Paleo diet.
- My clothes were looser. My shirts and pants that were too tight to wear are now comfortable and I can breathe in them.
- My skin improved. Before starting the Whole30, I had acne and oily skin, and huge pores. By the end of the 30 days, my skin appears clearer, brighter, and my acne is gone.
- After the first week, I have more energy than usual. I'm not tired after work and I genuinely look forward to exercising.
- I don't hate myself after meals. I used to feel terrible and guilty after eating anything and this stressed me out and would find something to eat to cope with the stress.
- I don't hate myself after meals anymore. I used to feel terrible and guilty after eating anything and this stressed me out. Because of the stress, I would find something else to eat just to cope. After the Whole30, I feel lighter, cleaner, happier, and prouder of myself after meals.

I'm so proud of myself after realizing that I had the power to turn my life around for the better. My eating habits and lifestyle are much healthier and better than ever before. It really does begin with your relationship with food!

My life has changed thanks to the Whole30 program and I can guarantee that your life will change too after a successful Whole30.

I hope that this book will provide you with everything you need to succeed!

Chapter 1: The Whole30 Diet

In this chapter, you will learn everything you need to know about the Whole30 Diet, which includes:

- What is the Whole30 Diet?
- Benefits of the Whole30
- Whole30 Shopping List
- Whole30 Foods to Avoid
- Rules of the Whole30 Program
- How to Get Started on the Whole30?
- Tips for Surviving the Whole30 Diet
- What to Do After the Whole30
- Whole30 FAQ

What is the Whole30 Diet?

The average person eats too much-processed foods these days. Busy people tend to eat more commercially manufactured drinks, meals, and snacks during the week. When unrestrained, these unhealthy eating habits lead to unintentional weight gain, and many chronic illnesses influenced by an imbalanced diet and a sluggish lifestyle.

Unhealthy eating habits plus little or no exercise have been accused as major contributors to lifelong illnesses and shortened life expectancy. Luckily for you, in the Whole30 diet, you can reset your system by adding more Whole Foods to your diet and cutting your daily intake of processed food and drinks for at least 30.

There are so many diets to choose from on how to be healthy – from veganism to the ketogenic diet, to weight-watchers, to the Atkins diet but the Whole30 diet is especially special as the sole purpose of the diet is to reset your system and to reevaluate your relationship with food.

The Whole30 is a revolutionary diet that can reset your relationship with food. The philosophy is to strictly restrict certain products without keeping track of calories and without recording the weight on the scale. The Whole30 diet is meant to be followed for at least 30 before you see and feel the benefit, and in most cases, those who successfully follow the Whole30 for a month tend to stick with the diet even further. The food groups that are cut out from the Whole30 are listed below:

- No grains are allowed on the Whole30
- No legumes are allowed on the Whole30
- No alcohol in any form is allowed on the Whole30
- No dairy is allowed on the Whole30
- No sugar in any form is allowed on the Whole30
- No MSG, sulfites, and carrageenan is allowed on the Whole30

The main rule for a successful Whole30 is to make sure you don't consume any food items from the groups listed above.

Benefits of the Whole30

Why should you or anyone else follow a Whole30 diet? Well, there's a huge list of benefits of Whole30 diet, the major benefits include the following:

- **Clearer and brighter skin, healthy fingernails and healthy hair:** Once you start to cut down unhealthy and processed foods from your diet, the appearance and condition of your skin, fingernails, and hair will improve drastically.
- **Increased energy:** It has been suggested that the Whole30 can triple a person's energy. This is because you are fueling your body with 100% pure natural energy. However, this increased in energy is not going to happen instantly. You will feel tired and lack energy during the first week of the Whole30, but after your body adjusts itself to the Whole30 diet, you soon will feel a boost in energy.
- **The Whole30 will help you lose weight:** Since you are getting rid of sugar, dairy, wheat, and junk food from your diet it will certainly help burn some fat.
- **Improve the quality of sleep:** The Whole30 has been proven to help to improve and to regulate the hormones in your body. This helps with how your body sleeps and improve your sleeping patterns.
- **Mental clarity and better focus:** When you are consuming whole foods, fresh meats, and organic vegetables it will help you stay healthy, focused, and energized throughout the day.
- **The Whole30 can help fight certain diseases:** Multiple diseases such as diabetes, cerebral palsy, or certain psychological disorders can be eliminated while being on a Whole30 diet. Patients with such diseases and disorders have shown an improvement from these chronic diseases while on the Whole30 diet.

Whole30 Shopping List

The Whole30 Diet is easy to follow. You just need to follow the Whole Food rules for 30 days with zero cheat days.

Below you will find a fully comprehensive list of delicious Whole Foods that are unprocessed or minimally processed that you can enjoy without guilt during the month-long challenge. Each recipe in this book is fully compliant with these rules and they can all be enjoyed throughout the Whole Food 30-day challenge and beyond.

Stock your refrigerator and pantry by grocery shopping with the full Whole30 Shopping List below:

Vegetables: All vegetables are allowed on the Whole30 Diet – including potatoes! Here's a full list of all the encouraged vegetables in the Whole30:

- Potatoes
- Asparagus
- Green beans
- Romaine lettuce
- Broccoli
- Bell pepper

- Carrot
- Red bell pepper
- Tomatoes
- Olives
- Avocado
- Garlic
- Cabbage
- Cucumber
- Brussels sprout
- Iceberg lettuce
- Celery
- Spinach
- Onion
- Zucchini
- Jalapeno peppers
- Pumpkin
- Sweet potatoes
- Peas
- Artichoke
- Mushrooms
- Kale
- Spinach
- Ginger
- Beets
- Eggplants
- Collard greens
- Chives
- Fennel
- Okra
- Leeks
- Radishes

Meat and Poultry: Unprocessed meat and poultry are allowed on the Whole30, but make sure you be on the lookout for added sugars and processed meats. Go shopping for these kinds of meat and poultry:

- Beef
- Ground beef
- Beef heart
- Beef Liver
- Beef tongue
- Buffalo, bison
- Goat
- Rabbit
- Mutton
- Chicken
- Lamb
- Pork
- Ham
- Ribs
- Pork shoulder
- Veal
- Bacon
- Burger
- Duck
- Duck Liver
- Chicken liver
- Turkey
- Quail
- Pheasant
- Sausage Patties
- Hotdog
- Bratwursts

Fruits: Both fresh and dried fruits are allowed on the Whole30, this includes:

- Bananas
- Apples
- Oranges
- Mangos
- Watermelon
- Pineapples
- Papaya
- Grapefruit
- Pomegranate
- Pear
- Peach
- Plum
- Grapes
- Kiwi
- Strawberries
- Blueberries
- Lemons
- Limes

Fish and Seafood: Fish and shellfish are encouraged in the Whole30 challenge. This includes:

- Tilapia
- Salmon
- Tuna
- Trout
- Black Cod
- Halibut
- Cod
- Catfish
- Barramundi
- Arctic char
- Crab
- Lobster
- Shrimp
- Clams
- Mussels
- Oysters
- Scallops

Fats: Fats is allowed on the Whole30, which include:

- Coconut oil
- Avocado oil
- Sesame oil
- Sunflower oil
- Canola oil
- Olive oil

- Ghee (clarified butter)
- Lard
- Duck fat
- Almond butter

Nuts and seeds: All nuts and seeds are encouraged on the Whole30 with the exception of peanuts, this includes:

- Nut milk (almond milk, cashew milk, flax milk, hazelnut milk, etc.)
- Nut flours (almond flour, coconut flour, flaxseed meal, macadamia nut flour, pistachio flour, cashew nut flour, etc.)

- Almonds
- Cashews
- Chestnuts
- Pecans
- Walnuts
- Pine nuts
- Macadamia nuts
- Flaxseeds
- Sesame seeds
- Chia seeds
- Sunflower seeds
- Pumpkin seeds

Note: Be extra attentive when checking the nut milk as they can contain hidden sugars, which is restricted from the Whole30.

Vinegar: Vinegar is allowed on the Whole30 diet, this includes:

- White vinegar
- Red wine vinegar
- Balsamic vinegar
- Apple cider vinegar

Herbs and seasonings: To enhance the flavors of your meal there are no restrictions on seasonings, spices, and herbs.

Whole30 Foods to Avoid

The Whole30 has a list of foods that are restricted. It's extremely important you don't have any cheat days or sneak in any of these foods in your meals for a successful Whole30.

Dairy: Dairy is not recommended on the Whole30, whether its full-fat or low-fat, the only exception of dairy allowed on the Whole30 is ghee, items to avoid include:

- Butter
- Milk
- Whey, milk powder
- Ice cream
- Frozen desserts
- Yogurt
- Soy and soy products
- Cottage cheese
- Sour cream
- Dips
- Natural and processed cheese
- Butter
- Non-dairy coffee creamer

Alcohol: No alcohol in any form is allowed on the Whole30 whether it's for cooking or drinking, this includes:

- Beer
- Tequila
- Vodka
- Gin
- Rum
- Vanilla extract

Note: The closest thing to alcohol on the Whole30 is cooking vinegar such as red wine vinegar, white vinegar, apple cider vinegar, etc.

Grains: All grains must be avoided, this includes:

- Rice
- Quinoa
- Oats
- Barley
- Maze
- Wheat

- Millet
- Farro
- Rye
- Buckwheat
- Spelt

Legumes: Legumes must be avoided on the Whole30, the only exceptions are peas and green beans, avoid the following:

- Tofu
- Soy sauce
- Miso
- Edamame
- Chickpeas
- Lentils
- Peanuts

Sugar and sweeteners: Sugar of any form is absolutely restricted on the Whole30. This includes sweeteners such as Swerve, Splenda, etc.

Processed additives: Any foods that contain MSG, carrageenan, or sulfites must be avoided.

Rules of the Whole30 Diet

The three general rules to follow on the Whole30 diet are:

1. No cheating
2. No recreating unhealthy options
3. No stepping on the scale or measuring your body
4. Avoid certain food groups

No cheating on the Whole30

To get the most out of the Whole30 program, it is highly recommended that you don't cheat. The Whole30 is all-or-nothing, so plan ahead – especially if it's around holidays, birthdays, traveling or socializing where you have no control over any available foods and drinks.

If you are a busy person, it's a good idea to have prepared meals in advance. Meals such as soups, stews, and salads can be stored in your refrigerator until ready to eat.

Don't recreate unhealthy foods or drinks.

Many people think that recreating a Whole30 cheesecake is fine as long as the ingredients are Whole30 compliant.

However, you must avoid recreating unhealthy food and drinks even if you are using Whole30 compliant ingredients. This can contribute to unintentional weight gain, physical illness, mental illness, and phycological disorders. Trying to recreate unhealthy food into healthy ones will defeat the purpose of the Whole30, and will only waste your time, energy, and money.

My advice for you is to keep an open mind about new recipes and ingredients. If you restrict yourself to a few meals, you will quickly tire out your taste buds and your patience. Luckily for you, in this book, you will find a diverse set of recipes that you can enjoy each day.

Don't weight yourself

Daily weighing in and measuring your body is not allowed on the Whole30. The Whole30 diet encourages gradual and safe weight loss. You're not going to find any dramatic change in your weight if you check the scale each day. Instead, weigh and measure yourself before and after the Whole30 diet.

Avoid certain food items

The main rule of the Whole30 diet is to not consume any items from the following food groups:

- Any form of alcohol
- Any form of sugar or sweetener
- Any form of baked goods such as cakes, cupcakes, cheesecakes, cookies
- Dairy
- Processed foods
- Junk food
- Candies and sweets
- Pasta
- Grains
- Starchy foods
- Instant gravy mixes and sauces
- Processed Meats
- Legumes
- Processed snacks

You will find a fully comprehensive list in the "Whole30 Foods to Avoid" section.

How to Get Started on the Whole30 Diet

Starting the Whole30 diet can feel daunting. Luckily for you, here you will learn how to get started on the Whole30 and successfully stick with it. Here is how you can get started:

Stock your pantry, refrigerator, and kitchen with Whole30 compliant foods: The first step is to get rid of all the food items that are not allowed on the Whole30 – this will make the challenge much easier and less likely for you to break any rules. After you get rid of all the bad foods, you need to go grocery shopping and start stocking on the following:

- Healthy cooking oil
- Meats
- Fish and seafood
- Lots of vegetables
- Fruit
- Plenty of water

Make a commitment: After you stock your kitchen with Whole30 foods you must make a commitment to yourself. Commit yourself to the Whole30 challenge and promise that you won't break any of the Whole30 general rules.

Meal plan: Finally, you must only make sure you eat Whole30 safe meals. To make your life easier, you can find a 30-day Whole Foods meal plan in Chapter 4.

Tips for Surviving the Whole30 Diet

Adopting a new diet can be difficult. However, with these tips, you can certainly survive the Whole30 diet for a month and beyond.

Make sure you get enough sleep: Sleep is often an underestimated in the Whole30. However, sleep is crucial as it allows your body to heal. Your metabolism and sleep are controlled by the same centers of your brain. Sleep deprivation can lead to weight gain. Do your best to improve your quality of sleep, and you will certainly feel better and motivated on the Whole30.

Drink enough water: Water is the most essential substance in your body so you must remain hydrated. Make sure that you drink 8 to 10 glasses of water daily and remain well hydrated during the 30-days. Drinking enough water allows your liver to break down fats more effectively. In the Whole30, you most likely will need additional water to make up for caffeinated beverages you eliminated from your diet.

Exercise: To meet your Whole30 goals, exercising is important. Exercising helps increases muscle functions and reduces the fat content in your body. You can choose between cardio, strength, or flexibility exercises which can give you enough physical activity daily to improve and maintain a healthy body.

Add more vegetables to your meals: Adding vegetables to your meals increases the nutritious value. For instance, eat vegetables as sides or as part of the main entrée. Examples include:

- Add spinach, onions, and herbs into egg omelets
- Puree carrots or other vegetables into smoothies
- Mix cauliflower or broccoli into scrambled eggs
- Try butternut squash pancakes with maple butter rather than regular flour pancakes.
- Add zucchini or spinach to homemade brownies
- Add extra vegetables to soups and stews
- Serve your favorite vegetables along with chicken, beef, pork, and fish recipes.

Substitute foods: You can adopt the Whole30 better by whole foods in place of processed foods. Such examples include:

- Instead of tamari and soy sauce use coconut aminos
- Instead of all-purpose flour use coconut flour
- Use flax meal instead of breadcrumbs
- Instead of cow's milk use unsweetened coconut milk or almond milk
- Instead of using bread use lettuce leaves
- Instead of rice use cauliflower rice
- Fresh vegetables instead of canned vegetables
- Olive oil and vinegar instead of store-bought salad dressing and ranch
- Instead of pasta noodles use spiralized squash or zucchini
- Instead of branded yogurt try unsweetened, plain Greek yogurt with fruit
- Frozen unsweetened smoothies instead of ice cream

Plan your meals: During the Whole30 challenge, you might become tired and don't feel like cooking anything, especially since whole foods are more time consuming than processed and packaged dishes. The answer is to plan your meals. This can mean doing all the food preparation for the recipe until dinnertime comes or have a simple lettuce salad stored in your refrigerator. Knowing what you are going to eat for what day can help you avoid cheating for a successful Whole30.

Be prepared for mistakes: You aren't a robot who can just be reprogrammed to eat only whole foods, don't expect a successful Whole30 without making any mistakes. You may accidentally eat or drink something you shouldn't have and you must be prepared to forgive yourself then. Being prepared for mistakes will make you feel less guilty when you drink a can of Coca-Cola or eat that chocolate chip cookie.

Find an accountability partner: Some people cannot motivate themselves in the Whole30 alone. The Whole30 encourages support and validation from other peoples, whether it's from friends, family, or fellow Whole30 dieters. It can be reassuring to know that you can talk to someone when you're having a tough day on the Whole30 and someone who understands the challenges you are facing.

What to Do After Whole30?

You've spent the entire month on whole foods, meal prepping, snacking less, no sweets, and reading nutrition labels thoroughly for hidden sugars. But now that the 30 days on Whole30 is over, you're probably wondering what do you do next?

There are many cases of people who've successfully finished the Whole30, gained an increase in energy, lost weight, and relapsed to their old eating habits. This means that the Whole30 is not a diet you can sustain your entire life.

It's not rocket science to suggest that if you relapse back to your old unhealthy habits – skipping meals, eating too much sugar, drinking alcohol, neglecting sleep and water – then you're not going to be healthy.

The Whole30 was created for individuals to reevaluate their relationship with food and make lifelong changes and habits that are highly individualized and sustainable to every person.

So, after a month of the whole30, think about how your life improved by eliminating certain groups. For example, your stomach issues may have disappeared after you cut out gluten or dairy. Or maybe your skin cleared up after you stopped consuming sugar.

Be carefully attentive of how you reintroduce certain foods to your diet. It is advised that you add one food to your diet and after a couple of days move onto the next one. Using this method, you will be able to identify what foods irritate you the most, and you can decide if you want to eliminate it permanently life after Whole30

So, to answer the question what to do after the Whole30, here are some ideas:

- Rethink your current diet: Decide whether you want to add dairy, sugar, grains, legumes back to your diet or stick to only eating whole foods.
- Think about next time: You can always turn to the Whole30 at any time if you feel like you aren't living your life as amazing as it was while on the Whole30 challenge.
- Live your life: One major downfall of the Whole30 is simply reverting to your unhealthy old eating habits. Rather than incorporating unhealthy junk food back into your diet, try to only have 1 to 2 weeks per week where you can enjoy any fun foods you like.

Whole30 FAQ

Here you will find frequently asked questions and answers regarding the Whole30. Refer to this section whenever you have a question during the diet.

What is the Whole30?

The Whole30 is a diet where you eliminate certain food groups from your diet for 30 days in an effort to reset your body and reevaluate your relationship with food.

What can I eat during the Whole30?

You can eat real whole food such as meat, seafood, eggs, vegetables, fruit, fats, oils, nuts, and seeds. Natural, unprocessed and organic food is heavily encouraged on the Whole30.

What can I not eat during the Whole30?

For 30-days you cannot eat any forms of sugar or sweetener, alcohol, grains, dairy, legumes, and any food that contains carrageenan, MSG or sulfites.

Will I lose weight on the Whole30?

Most people on the Whole30 will lose weight, but the sole purpose of the Whole30 is not to lose weight but to remove foods and food groups that negatively affect your health.

Can the Whole30 cure diseases and illnesses?

Many people on the Whole30 claims that the Whole30 challenge helped prevent, improved, or cured illnesses such as:

- High blood pressure
- Type 1 Diabetes
- Type 2 diabetes
- High cholesterol
- Asthma
- Allergies
- Skin conditions
- Infertility
- Bipolar disorders
- Depression
- Leaky gut syndrome
- Joint pain and other illnesses

What are some benefits that come with the Whole30?

There are many physical benefits that come with the Whole30, which includes:

- Improved body composition/posture
- Improved energy levels
- Better sleep quality
- Better attention span
- Better athletic performance

Psychological benefits of the Whole30 challenge include:

- Reduction or elimination of food cravings, sugar, and carbs
- New healthy habits
- Improved mental clarity
- Improved memory
- Improved self-confidence

Can I have a cheat day during the Whole30 challenge?
No, for a successful Whole30 diet you must be strict not to eat any "cheat" or "junk" foods. Zero exceptions.

Can I adjust the Whole30 diet?
No one is forcing you to not eat the restricted foods, however, you may not experience all the benefits after the 30-days are up.

Can I make cupcakes, cakes, or "junk" food if I only use Whole30 allowed ingredients?
According to the Whole30 program, no, the Whole30 is designed to reevaluate your relationship with food in a healthy manner. Desserts, junk food, and sweets, even if only prepared with Whole30 allowed ingredients, is heavily discouraged.

If I mess up, do I have to reset back to day one?
Most of the time, yes. If you ate birthday cake, drink alcohol, or something sugary you should think about restarting the Whole30 challenge.

What if I am vegan?
Meat is highly encouraged on the Whole30, but you can still have a successful Whole30 by incorporating Whole30 compliant vegan sources such as nuts and seeds.

Chapter 2: 30-Day Whole Food Meal Plan

In this chapter, you will find a very effective Whole30 meal plan that will last you 30 days. This 30-day meal plan gives you loads of options to choose from for each day. Feel free to adjust the meal plan and anything on the menu depending on your preference.

Day 1
Meal one: Mythical Sweet and Sour Cabbage
Meal two: Gratifying Coconut Tomato Basil Soup
Meal three: Extremely Popular Red Wine Pot Roast with Winter Vegetables
Day 2
Meal one: Delightful Fish Tacos
Meal two: Magnificent Coconut Custard
Meal three: Packed with Flavor Mushroom Chicken Stroganoff
Day 3
Meal one: Heavenly Cream of Mushroom Lamb with Cauliflower Risotto
Meal two: Deliciously Acclaimed Broccoli and Sweet Potato Soup
Meal three: Worldwide Famous Whole30 Chili
Day 4
Meal one: Delicious Lemon Salmon Fillets with Garlic
Meal two: Celebrated Stuffed Pepper Soup
Meal three: Enjoyable Teriyaki Pork Tenderloin
Day 5
Meal one: Fiery Tuna Salad with Jalapeno
Meal two: Effortless Banana Custard
Meal three: Perfect Chicken with Red Beets and Fresh Artichokes
Day 6
Meal one: Grandmother's Garden Chicken Soup
Meal two: Yummy Greek Chicken
Meal three: Yawning Mashed Cauliflower
Day 7
Meal one: Family Favorite Creole Seafood Gumbo
Meal two: Wonderful Sautéed Swiss Chard with Nuts and Bacon
Meal three: Superstar Mushroom and Steak Stroganoff
Day 8
Meal one: Mythical Sweet and Sour Cabbage
Meal two: Beautiful Cinnamon Apple Slices
Meal three: Millionaire Beef and Broccoli
Day 9
Meal one: Well-Known Portuguese-Inspired Kale Soup
Meal two: One of the Kind Mashed Garlic Sweet Potatoes
Meal three: Unstoppable Pulled Pork with Whole30 Friendly Barbecue Sauce
Day 10

Meal one: Perfect Chicken with Red Beets and Fresh Artichokes
Meal two: Healthy and Delicious Borscht
Meal three: Intriguing Mediterranean Goat Roast with Sweet Potato and Vegetables
Day 11
Meal one: Full Body Cleansing Vegetable Soup
Meal two: Appetizing Herb-Buttered Carrots
Meal three: Unstoppable Pulled Pork with Whole30 Friendly Barbecue Sauce
Day 12
Meal one: Perfectly Steamed Mussels
Meal two: Glorious Brussel Sprouts with Pecans
Meal three: Highly Seasoned Barbacoa Beef Pot Roast
Day 13
Meal one: Extremely Delicious Chicken Shawarma
Meal two: Everyday Sautéed Peaches and Apples
Meal three: Summer Jamaican-Inspired Goat Curry
Day 14
Meal one: Pleasant Bacon-Wrapped Asparagus
Meal two: Enchanting Sautéed Garlic Artichokes
Meal three: Fashionable Pork Steaks with Cremini Mushrooms, Sweet Potatoes, and Gravy
Day 15
Meal one: Healthy and Delicious Borscht
Meal two: Welcoming Sautéed Lemon-Garlic Kale
Meal three: Overpowering Pressure-Cooked Balsamic Rosemary Lamb Chops
Day 16
Meal one: One of the Kind Mashed Garlic Sweet Potatoes
Meal two: Hearty Spaghetti Squash Cauliflower Alfredo
Meal three: Happy Hawaiian-Inspired Pork
Day 17
Meal one: Delicious Lemon Salmon Fillets with Garlic
Meal two: Welcoming Sautéed Lemon-Garlic Kale
Meal three: Flavorful Mediterranean Style Fish
Day 18
Meal one: Crowd-Pleasing Buffalo Chicken Dip
Meal two: You Will Love These Vegan Stuffed Bell Peppers
Meal three: Extremely Popular Red Wine Pot Roast with Winter Vegetables
Day 19
Meal one: Wonderful Sautéed Swiss Chard with Nuts and Bacon
Meal two: Hearty Spaghetti Squash Cauliflower Alfredo
Meal three: Celebrated Stuffed Pepper Soup
Day 20
Meal one: Flavorful Cauliflower Tikka Masala
Meal two: Beautiful Cinnamon Apple Slices
Meal three: Extraordinary Sesame Garlic Lamb
Day 21

Meal one: <u>Wicked Calamari with Tomato Sauce</u>
Meal two: <u>Victorious Chocolate Cupcakes</u>
Meal three: <u>Invincible Beef Roast with Whole30 BBQ and Coleslaw</u>
Day 22
Meal one: <u>Terrific Barbecue Lamb Meatloaf</u>
Meal two: <u>Fabulous Berry Compote</u>
Meal three: <u>Exciting Beef Ragu</u>
Day 23
Meal one: <u>Well-Done Moroccan Spiced Sweet Potatoes</u>
Meal two: <u>Full Body Cleansing Vegetable Soup</u>
Meal three: <u>Enjoyable Teriyaki Pork Tenderloin</u>
Day 24
Meal one: <u>Out of This World Bratwurst and Cabbage</u>
Meal two: <u>Welcoming Sautéed Lemon-Garlic Kale</u>
Meal three: <u>Grand Chicken Cacciatore</u>
Day 25
Meal one: <u>Celebrated Sweet Potato Soup</u>
Meal two: <u>Nicest Homemade Caramel-Applesauce</u>
Meal three: <u>Lovely Cuban-Inspired Garlicky Pork</u>
Day 26
Meal one: <u>Enchanting Sautéed Garlic Artichokes</u>
Meal two: <u>Well-Known Portuguese-Inspired Kale Soup</u>
Meal three: <u>Honorable Yukon Potato Curry</u>
Day 27
Meal one: <u>Pleasant Bacon-Wrapped Asparagus</u>
Meal two: <u>Perfect Banana Foster</u>
Meal three: <u>Exotic Vegan Chili</u>
Day 28
Meal one: <u>Exquisite Kale and Carrots with Bacon</u>
Meal two: <u>Heroic Creamy Cauliflower and Fennel Soup</u>
Meal three: <u>Award Winning Seafood Chili</u>
Day 29
Meal one: <u>You Will Love These Vegan Stuffed Bell Peppers</u>
Meal two: <u>Pleasurable and Healthy Green Chicken Soup</u>
Meal three: <u>Highly Seasoned Barbacoa Beef Pot Roast</u>
Day 30
Meal one: <u>Desirable Brussel Sprouts with Mango and Nuts</u>
Meal two: <u>Lovely Polish-Inspired Cabbage Soup</u>
Meal three: <u>Favorite Smooth Pumpkin Custard</u>

Just as a careful reminder, this is only a sample 4-week Whole30 meal plan that you can follow to get started with the challenge. Feel free to switch up the meal plan as long as it's Whole30 safe.

Chapter 3: Delicious Chicken and Poultry Recipes

Homemade Low-Sodium Chicken Stock

Time: 1 hour
Servings: 8 cups of chicken stock
Ingredients:

- 2 pounds of whole chicken (with pieces, skin, bones, carcasses, feet, wings, etc.)
- 2 medium-sized fresh carrots, uncut and unpeeled
- 1 medium-sized onions, peeled and cut into 4 pieces
- 2 medium-sized fresh celery stalks, uncut and cleaned
- 4 parsley stalks
- A few sprigs of thyme
- 2 bay leaves
- 4 garlic cloves
- 8 cups of water

Instructions:

- Add all the ingredients to your Instant Pot.
- Lock the lid and ensure the valve is sealed. Press the "Manual" button and cook for40 minutes on High Pressure.
- When the timer beeps, allow for a full natural release before carefully removing the lid.
- Remove the contents of the Instant Pot and transfer the liquid to jars for future use.

Nutrition information per serving:

- Calories: 193
- Fat: 13.2g
- Carbohydrates: 2.5g
- Dietary Fiber: 0g
- Protein: 14.3g

Crowd-Pleasing Avocado Lime Chicken Soup

Time: 25 minutes
Servings: 6
Ingredients:

- 1 ½ pounds of fresh boneless, skinless chicken breasts or thighs
- 1 tablespoon of coconut oil
- 4 cups of homemade low-sodium chicken stock
- 2 garlic cloves, minced
- 2 medium-sized green jalapeno peppers, seeded and finely chopped
- 3 large tomatoes, finely chopped
- 1 cup of finely chopped green onions
- 4 medium-sized ripe avocados, peeled and cut into pieces
- 4 fresh radishes, sliced into pieces
- ½ cup of unsweetened coconut cream
- 1 teaspoon of ground cumin
- 1 teaspoon of dried oregano
- 1 teaspoon of sea salt (to taste)
- 1 teaspoon of freshly ground black pepper (to taste)
- 1 teaspoon of ground coriander powder
- 1/3 cup of fresh cilantro, finely chopped
- 3 tablespoons of fresh lime juice

Instructions:

- Press the "Sauté" function on your Instant Pot and add the olive oil.
- Once the display reads hot, add the green onions and jalapeno peppers. Sauté for 3 softened or until softened.
- Add the garlic and sauté for an extra minute.
- Add the chicken stock, chicken breasts or thighs, tomatoes, ground cumin, dried oregano, salt, black pepper, and coriander powder to your Instant Pot.
- Lock the lid and ensure the valve is closed. Press the "Manual" button and cook for 10 minutes on High Pressure.
- When the cooking is done, naturally release the pressure and remove the lid.
- Stir in the radishes and transfer the chicken to a serving platter.
- Shred the chicken using two forks and return to your Instant Pot.
- Stir in the lime juice, cilantro, avocados, and unsweetened coconut cream.
- Serve and enjoy!

Nutrition information per serving:

- Calories: 145
- Fat: 13g
- Carbohydrates: 5.3g
- Dietary Fiber: 0.9g
- Protein: 14.5g

Perfect Chicken with Red Beets and Fresh Artichokes

Time: 23 minutes
Servings: 4
Ingredients:

- 4 bone-in, skin on chicken breasts, thighs, or drumsticks
- 1 medium-sized red onion, finely chopped
- 6 garlic cloves, minced
- 2 tablespoons of coconut oil, olive oil, or avocado oil
- 1 fresh lemon, juice and zest
- 1 cup of homemade low-sodium chicken stock
- 1 medium-sized red beet, peeled and chopped
- ½ cup of Kalamata olives, pitted and sliced
- 6 fresh medium-sized artichoke hearts, finely chopped
- 1 tablespoon of fresh parsley leaves, finely chopped
- 1 teaspoon of sea salt (to taste)
- 1 teaspoon of freshly ground black pepper (to taste)

Instructions:

- Season the chicken with salt and black pepper
- Press the "Sauté" function on your Instant Pot and add the coconut oil or olive oil.
- Once hot, add the chicken and sauté for 2 to 4 minutes per side or until golden brown. Remove and set aside.
- Add the onion and garlic to your Instant Pot. Sauté for 4 minutes or until lightly browned, stirring occasionally.
- Return the chicken to your Instant Pot and add the lemon zest, lemon juice, chicken stock, chopped beet, and chopped artichoke hearts to your Instant Pot.
- Lock the lid and ensure the valve is closed on your Instant Pot. Press the "Manual" button and cook for 12 minutes on High Pressure.
- When the cooking is done, naturally release the pressure and remove the lid.
- Stir in the Kalamata olives and parsley.
- Check if the chicken is cooked through and if the vegetables are softened. Adjust the seasoning as needed.
- Serve and enjoy!

Nutrition information per serving:

- Calories: 212
- Fat: 6.8g
- Carbohydrates: 3.3g
- Dietary Fiber: 0.4g
- Protein: 32.5g

Family-Oriented Whole30 Balsamic Chicken with Veggies

Time: 25 minutes
Servings: 6
Ingredients:

- 1 ½ pounds of fresh boneless, skinless chicken breasts or thighs
- 2 tablespoons of olive oil or coconut oil
- 1 cup of Portobello mushrooms, sliced
- 1 cup of green beans, trimmed and cut
- 2 medium-sized orange carrots, peeled and cut
- 3 medium-sized celery stalks, cut into pieces
- 1 medium-sized red bell pepper, deseeded and chopped
- 1 medium-sized green bell pepper, deseeded and chopped
- 4 garlic cloves, minced
- 1 medium-sized red onions, finely chopped
- 1 cup of homemade low sodium chicken broth
- 2 to 3 tablespoons of balsamic vinegar
- 1 tablespoon of fresh thyme
- 1 tablespoon of fresh parsley, finely chopped
- 1 teaspoon of sea salt (to taste)
- 1 teaspoon of freshly ground black pepper (to taste)

Instructions:

- Season the chicken with salt and pepper.
- Press the "Sauté" function on your Instant Pot and add the olive oil.
- Once the display reads hot, add the chicken and sauté on both sides for 2 minutes or until brown. Remove and set aside.
- Add the onion, garlic, mushrooms, green beans, and bell peppers to your Instant Pot and sauté for 3 minutes or until softened, stirring occasionally.
- Return the chicken to your Instant Pot. Add the chicken broth, parsley, balsamic vinegar, and thyme to your Instant Pot and stir until well combined.
- Lock the lid and ensure the valve is closed. Press the "Manual" button and cook for 8 minutes on High Pressure.
- When the cooking is done, naturally or quick release the pressure and remove the lid. Check if the chicken and vegetables are cooked.
- Serve and enjoy!

Nutrition information per serving:

- Calories: 255
- Fat: 8.6g
- Carbohydrates: 9.5g
- Dietary Fiber: 2.3g
- Protein: 34.6g

Charming Chicken Tikka Masala

Time: 30 minutes
Servings: 4
Ingredients:

- 1 ½ pounds of boneless, skinless chicken breasts
- ½ cup of homemade low sodium chicken stock
- ½ cup of unsweetened coconut milk
- 1 lemon, juice
- 1 tablespoon of fresh basil, chopped
- 1 tablespoon of fresh cilantro, chopped
- 2 tablespoons of extra virgin olive oil
- 3 garlic cloves, minced
- 1 small yellow onion, finely chopped
- 1 1-inch piece of ginger, peeled and grated
- 1 tablespoon of paprika
- 1 teaspoon of garam masala
- 1 teaspoon of organic ground turmeric
- 2 teaspoons of organic ground cumin
- 1 teaspoon of organic ground coriander
- ¼ teaspoon of organic cayenne pepper
- ¼ teaspoon of crushed red pepper flakes
- 1 teaspoon of sea salt
- 1 teaspoon of freshly ground black pepper
- 1 tablespoon of almond flour
- 1 (14-ounce) can of diced tomatoes, undrained

Instructions:

- Press the "Sauté" function on your Instant Pot and add the olive oil.
- Once the display reads hot, add the garlic, ginger, and onions to your Instant Pot. Sauté for 4 minutes or until lightly browned, stirring occasionally.
- Add all the spices and seasonings to your Instant Pot and stir until well combined.
- Stir in the tomatoes to your Instant Pot.
- Place the chicken on top of the tomatoes and add the chicken stock.
- Lock the lid and ensure the valve is closed. Press the "Manual" button and cook for 7 minutes on High Pressure.
- When the cooking is done, quick release the pressure and remove the lid.
- Transfer the chicken to a cutting board and cut into bite-sized pieces. Return the chicken to your Instant Pot.
- Press the "Sauté" function on your Instant Pot and allow to simmer for 4 minutes.
- Stir in the unsweetened coconut milk, lemon juice, and almond flour to your Instant Pot.
- Top with fresh basil and fresh cilantro. Serve and enjoy!

Nutrition information per serving:

- Calories: 429
- Fat: 20.1g
- Carbohydrates: 10.5g
- Dietary Fiber: 3g
- Protein: 51.7g

Irresistible Italian Chicken Meatballs

Time: 40 minutes
Servings: 4
Chicken Meatball Ingredients:

- 1 pound of lean ground chicken
- 1 large egg
- 1 tablespoon of coconut oil
- 1 tablespoon of coconut or almond flour
- 2 tablespoons of fresh basil, finely chopped
- 1 teaspoon of salt
- 1 teaspoon of black pepper

Vegetable Ingredients:

- ½ tablespoon of coconut oil
- 1 large red bell pepper, deseeded and sliced
- 1 large bunch of asparagus, chopped
- 2 cups of green beans, chopped
- 1 cup of low sodium homemade chicken stock
- 1 cup of cherry tomatoes, halved

Instructions:

- In a large bowl, add all the chicken meatball ingredients besides the olive oil and stir until well combined.
- Form the mixture into meatballs and set aside.
- Press the "Sauté" function on your Instant Pot and add ½ tablespoon of coconut oil.
- Once the display reads hot, add the red bell pepper, asparagus, and green beans. Sauté for 3 minutes or until softened, stirring occasionally Remove and set aside.
- Add 1 tablespoon of coconut oil to your Instant Pot. Working in batches, add the meatballs and cook until brown.
- Add all the meatballs and vegetables to your Instant Pot. Add the chicken stock to your Instant Pot.
- Lock the lid and ensure the valve is closed.
- Press the "Manual" button and cook for 10 minutes on High Pressure.
- When the cooking is done, naturally release the pressure and remove the lid.
- Stir in the cherry tomato halves.
- Serve and enjoy!

Nutrition information per serving:

- Calories: 312
- Fat: 17.3g
- Carbohydrates: 9.5g
- Dietary Fiber: 4.1g
- Protein: 26.2g

Yummy Greek Chicken

Time: 33 minutes
Servings: 6
Ingredients:

- 2 pounds of boneless, skinless fresh chicken thighs
- 2 tablespoons of olive oil or avocado oil
- 3 garlic cloves, minced
- 1 teaspoon of dried oregano
- 1 teaspoon of dried thyme
- 1 teaspoon of dried parsley flakes
- 1 tablespoon of almond flour
- 1 tablespoon of fresh basil, finely chopped
- 1 teaspoon of sea salt (to taste)
- 1 teaspoon of freshly ground black pepper (to taste)
- 1 red onion, finely chopped
- 1 cup of Kalamata olives, sliced
- 1 cup of homemade low sodium chicken stock or plain water
- ¼ cup of red wine vinegar
- ½ lemon, juiced
- 1 to 2 tablespoons of almond flour
- 1 (12-ounce) jar of organic marinated fire roasted red peppers, drained and chopped
- 1 (8-ounce) jar of organic marinated artichoke hearts, drained

Instructions:

- Press the "Sauté" function on your Instant Pot and add the olive oil.
- Once the display reads hot, add the garlic and sauté for 1 minute or until fragrant, stirring occasionally.
- Add the chicken and cook for 2 minutes per side until brown.
- Add the marinated artichoke hearts, marinated peppers, and Kalamata olives to your Instant Pot. Top with red onion slices
- Add the chicken stock, red wine vinegar, lemon juice, oregano, parsley, and thyme to your Instant Pot.
- Lock the lid and ensure the valve is closed on your Instant Pot. Press the "Manual" button and cook for 7 minutes on High Pressure.
- When the cooking is done, naturally release or quick release the pressure and remove the lid.
- Press the "Sauté" function on your Instant Pot and sprinkle with almond flour. Allow to simmer until thickens. Serve and enjoy!

Nutrition information per serving:

- Calories: 443
- Fat: 35.6g
- Carbohydrates: 3.9g
- Dietary Fiber: 1.3g
- Protein: 26g

Extremely Delicious Chicken Shawarma

Time: 20 minutes

Servings: 8

Ingredients:

- 3 pounds of fresh boneless, skinless chicken breasts, thighs, or tenderloins, sliced into strips
- 1 cup of low sodium chicken stock
- 1 tablespoon of smoked paprika
- 1 teaspoon of ground allspice powder
- 1 teaspoon of chili powder
- ½ teaspoon of ground cinnamon powder
- 1 teaspoon of sea salt (to taste)
- 1 teaspoon of freshly ground black pepper (to taste)
- ½ teaspoon of organic cayenne pepper
- ½ teaspoon of organic crushed red pepper flakes
- 2 teaspoons of organic ground cumin
- 2 teaspoons of ground turmeric powder
- 1 tablespoon of dried parsley flakes
- 1 tablespoon of dried basil
- Homemade Whole30-friendly tahini sauce (for serving)

Instructions:

- In a bowl, add all the seasonings and mix well.
- Season the chicken strips with the seasoning mix until well coated.
- Add the chicken stock and chicken strips to your Instant Pot.
- Lock the lid and ensure the valve is sealed. Press the "Poultry" button and cook for 15 minutes on High Pressure.
- When the cooking is done, naturally release the pressure for 10 minutes, and then quick release the remaining pressure. Carefully remove the lid.
- Transfer the chicken to serving plates and drizzle with tahini sauce.
- Serve and enjoy!

Nutrition information per serving:

- Calories: 258
- Fat: 5.3g
- Carbohydrates: 0g
- Dietary Fiber: 0g
- Protein: 49.3g

Packed with Flavor Mushroom Chicken Stroganoff

Time: 26 minutes
Servings: 6
Ingredients:

- 2 pounds of fresh boneless, skinless chicken breasts, cut into bite-sized pieces
- 2 tablespoons of olive oil or coconut oil
- 2 tablespoons of almond flour
- 4 garlic cloves, minced
- 1 cup of Portobello mushrooms, sliced
- 1 cup of low sodium homemade chicken stock
- 2 tablespoons of coconut aminos
- 1 tablespoon of apple cider vinegar
- ½ cup of unsweetened coconut milk
- ½ teaspoon of cayenne pepper
- 1 teaspoon of onion powder
- 1 teaspoon of sea salt (to taste)
- 1 teaspoon of freshly ground black pepper (to taste)

Instructions:

- Coat your chicken pieces with 2 tablespoons of almond flour.
- Press the "Sauté" function on your Instant Pot and add the olive oil.
- Once the display reads hot, add the chicken pieces and sauté for 2 minutes per side or until almost brown.
- Add the mushrooms and garlic to your Instant Pot and turn off "Sauté" function.
- In a small bowl, add the coconut aminos, apple cider vinegar, and chicken stock. Pour the mixture over the chicken and mushrooms.
- Lock the lid and ensure the valve is closed.
- Press the "Manual" button and cook for 7 minutes on High Pressure.
- When the cooking is done, naturally release the pressure for 15 minutes and then quick release the remaining pressure. Carefully remove the lid.
- Press the "Sauté" function on your Instant Pot and stir in the unsweetened coconut milk, cayenne pepper, onion powder, salt, and black pepper Allow to simmer for 10 minutes or until creamy, stirring occasionally. Serve and enjoy!

Nutrition information per serving:

- Calories: 317
- Fat: 14.1g
- Carbohydrates: 1.5g
- Dietary Fiber: 0.6g
- Protein: 44.7g

Entertaining Chicken Pineapple Tacos

Time: 30 minutes

Servings: 6

Ingredients:

- 2 pounds of fresh boneless, skinless chicken breasts
- 1 medium-sized sweet onion, finely chopped
- ½ cup of pineapple juice
- 1 cup of fresh pineapple chunks
- 1 fresh poblano pepper, sliced
- 2 chipotle peppers in adobo, finely chopped
- 3 garlic cloves, minced
- 1 tablespoon of chili powder
- 1 tablespoon of paprika
- ½ teaspoon of ground cumin
- 1 teaspoon of sea salt (to taste)
- 1 teaspoon of freshly ground black pepper (to taste)
- Lettuce leaves (for serving)
- Diced tomatoes (for serving)
- Avocado slices (for serving)

Pineapple Salsa Ingredients:

- 1 cup of fresh pineapple chunks
- 1 fresh jalapeno, minced
- ¼ cup of fresh cilantro, finely chopped
- Juice from 1 fresh lime

Instructions:

- Season the chicken with the chili powder, paprika, ground cumin, salt, and black pepper.
- Add the seasoned chicken to your Instant Pot along with the onion, garlic, poblano pepper, chipotle peppers, pineapple juice, and pineapple chunks to your Instant Pot.
- Lock the lid and ensure the valve is closed. Press the "Manual" button and cook for 20 minutes on High Pressure.
- When the cooking is done, either naturally release or quick release the pressure. Carefully remove the lid.
- Remove the chicken and transfer to a serving platter. Shred using two forks. Return to your Instant Pot and stir with the cooked pineapple mixture.
- In a bowl, add all the pineapple salsa ingredients and stir until well combined.
- Stuff the shredded chicken to lettuce leaves and top with pineapple salsa, tomatoes, and avocado slices. Serve and enjoy!

Nutrition information per serving:

- Calories: 277
- Fat: 4.7g
- Carbohydrates: 12.3g
- Dietary Fiber: 1.3g
- Protein: 44.6g

Tempting Southwestern Chicken with Cream

Time: 15 minutes

Servings: 6

Ingredients:

- 2 pounds of fresh boneless, skinless chicken breasts or tenderloins
- 2 sweet medium-sized red bell peppers, deseeded and sliced
- 1 cup of homemade low-sodium chicken stock
- Juice from 1 fresh lime
- 1 tablespoon of almond flour
- ½ cup of unsweetened coconut cream
- 1 tablespoon of chili powder
- 1 tablespoon of smoked paprika or regular paprika
- 1 teaspoon of organic ground cumin
- 2 tablespoons of olive oil or coconut oil
- 1 teaspoon of organic ground turmeric powder
- 1 teaspoon of garlic powder
- 1 teaspoon of onion powder
- 1 teaspoon of cayenne pepper
- ¼ cup of fresh cilantro, finely chopped (for garnishing)
- 1 teaspoon of sea salt (to taste)
- 1 teaspoon of freshly ground black pepper (to taste)

Instructions:

- In a small bowl, add the chili powder, paprika, cumin, garlic powder, onion powder, turmeric powder, salt, and black pepper.
- Season the chicken with half of the seasoning combination.
- Press the "Sauté" function on your Instant Pot and add the olive oil.
- Once the display reads hot, add the chicken and sauté until lightly browned.
- Add the chicken stock, juice from 1 lime, bell peppers, and remaining seasoning mixture to your Instant Pot.
- Lock the lid and ensure the valve is closed. Press the "Manual" button and cook for 7 minutes on High Pressure.
- When the cooking is done, quick release the pressure and carefully remove the lid.
- Gently stir in the unsweetened coconut cream and sprinkle with almond flour. Allow to cook until thick and creamy, stirring occasionally. Adjust the seasoning if necessary. Serve and enjoy!

Nutrition information per serving:

- Calories: 278
- Fat: 9.6g
- Carbohydrates: 1.3g
- Dietary Fiber: 0.5g
- Protein: 44.4g

Legendary Chicken Sweet Potato Curry

Time: 23 minutes
Servings: 6
Ingredients:

* 1 pounds of fresh boneless, skinless chicken breasts, cut into bite-sized pieces
* 2 cups of medium-sized sweet potatoes, peeled and cut into cubes
* 1 medium-sized red bell pepper, deseeded and either chopped or sliced
* 2 cups of fresh green beans, trimmed
* 1 cup of homemade low-sodium chicken stock
* 1 ¾ cup of unsweetened coconut milk
* ¼ cup of fresh cilantro, finely chopped
* 4 garlic cloves, minced
* ½ medium-sized yellow onions, finely chopped
* 1 tablespoon of coconut oil
* 3 tablespoons of curry powder
* 1 teaspoon of ground organic cumin
* 1 teaspoon of organic ground turmeric powder
* 1 teaspoon of cayenne pepper powder
* 1 teaspoon of sea salt (to taste)

Instructions:

* Press the "Sauté" function on your Instant Pot and add the coconut oil.
* Once the display reads hot, add the onions and garlic. Sauté for 4 minutes or until translucent, stirring occasionally. Turn off "Sauté" function on your Instant Pot.
* Add the 1 pound of fresh chicken pieces, 2 cups of sweet potatoes, 1 red bell pepper, 2 cups of green beans, 1 cup of chicken stock and all the seasonings to your Instant Pot.
* Lock the lid and ensure the valve is closed. Press the "Manual" button and cook for 12 minutes on High Pressure.
* When the cooking is done, quick release the pressure and carefully remove the lid.
* Press the "Sauté" function on your Instant Pot and gently stir in the unsweetened coconut milk.
* Ladle the curry into serving bowls and top with fresh cilantro
* Serve and enjoy!

Nutrition information per serving:

* Calories: 328
* Fat: 17g
* Carbohydrates: 13.3g
* Dietary Fiber: 3.9g
* Protein: 26.7g

Perfect Almond and Pear Chicken Wraps

Time: 20 minutes
Servings: 4
Chicken Ingredients:

- 2 pounds of fresh boneless, skinless chicken thighs
- 2 tablespoons of olive oil or coconut oil
- 1 cup of low-sodium chicken stock or ordinary water
- 1 teaspoon of salt
- 1 teaspoon of freshly ground black pepper

Salad Wrap Ingredients:

- 2 fresh romaine lettuce heads
- 1 fresh medium-sized pear, cored and finely chopped
- 1 tablespoon of fish sauce
- 1 fresh medium-sized lime, squeezed for juice
- 2 medium-sized orange carrots, finely grated
- 1 tablespoon of white vinegar
- ¼ cup of almond butter

Instructions:

- Season the chicken thighs with salt and black pepper.
- Press the "Sauté" function on your Instant Pot and add the olive oil.
- Once the display reads hot, add the chicken thighs and sauté for 4 minutes per side or until brown.
- Add the 1 cup of chicken stock to your Instant Pot.
- Place and seal the lid on your Instant Pot. Press the "Manual" button and cook for 5 minutes on High Pressure.
- When the cooking is done, naturally release the pressure for 5 minutes, then quick release the remaining pressure. Carefully remove the lid and transfer the chicken to a serving platter.
- Shred the chicken using two forks.
- In a large bowl, add the shredded chicken, pear, fish sauce, lime juice, grated carrot, white vinegar, and almond butter. Stir until well combined.
- Spoon the shredded chicken salad onto the romaine lettuce heads and tightly wrap together. Serve and enjoy!

Nutrition information per serving:

- Calories: 465
- Fat: 14.8g
- Carbohydrates: 13.5g
- Dietary Fiber: 3g
- Protein: 67.3g

Grand Chicken Cacciatore

Time: 27 minutes
Servings: 6
Ingredients:

- 2 pounds of boneless, skinless fresh chicken breasts
- 2 tablespoons of olive oil or coconut oil
- 1 medium-sized yellow onion, finely chopped
- 3 garlic cloves, minced
- 1 large-sized green bell pepper, deseeded and chopped
- 1 cup of mushrooms, sliced
- ½ cup of marinated artichoke hearts, finely chopped
- 1 cup of homemade low sodium chicken stock
- 1 (14-ounce) can of diced tomatoes, undrained
- ¼ cup of fresh tomato paste
- ¼ cup of red wine vinegar
- 1 teaspoon of dried oregano
- 1 teaspoon of dried thyme
- 1 teaspoon of dried rosemary
- 1 teaspoon of dried parsley flakes
- 1 teaspoon of smoked paprika
- 1 teaspoon of sea salt (to taste)
- 1 teaspoon of freshly ground black pepper (to taste)

Instructions:

- Season the chicken with salt and black pepper.
- Press the "Sauté" function on your Instant Pot and add the olive oil.
- Once the display reads hot, add the chicken and sauté until brown on each side. Remove and set aside.
- Add onions and garlic to your Instant Pot. Sauté for 2 minutes or until lightly browned, stirring occasionally. Turn off "Sauté" function.
- Return the chicken and add the remaining ingredients to your Instant Pot.
- Lock the lid and ensure the valve is closed. Press the "Manual" button and cook for 8 minutes on High Pressure.
- When the cooking is done, quick release the pressure and remove the lid.
- Give the chicken cacciatore a good stir and adjust the seasoning as needed.
- Serve and enjoy!

Nutrition information per serving:

- Calories: 307
- Fat: 9.5g
- Carbohydrates: 8.1g
- Dietary Fiber: 2.4g
- Protein: 45.7g

To Die For Harissa Chicken

Time: 16 minutes
Servings: 6
Ingredients:

- 2 pounds of fresh boneless, skinless chicken breast
- 1 (12-ounce) jar of organic fire roasted red peppers
- ½ fresh medium-sized lemon, juice
- 2 chipotle peppers in adobo sauce
- 1 medium red onion, finely chopped
- 4 garlic cloves, minced
- 2 tablespoons of olive oil
- ¼ cup of fresh cilantro, finely chopped
- 1 teaspoon of salt (to taste)
- 1 teaspoon of freshly ground black pepper (to taste
- 2 teaspoons of adobo sauce
- 1 tablespoon of apple cider vinegar
- 1 teaspoon of organic ground cumin
- 1 teaspoon of organic ground coriander powder
- ½ teaspoon of caraway seeds

Instructions:

- In a food processor, add the jar of fire roasted red peppers, 2 chipotle peppers, apple cider vinegar, lemon juice, salt, black pepper, adobo sauce, ground cumin, coriander powder, and caraway seeds. Pulse until smooth.
- Press the "Sauté" function on your Instant Pot and add the olive oil.
- Once the display reads hot, add the onion and sauté for 3 minutes or until browned, stirring occasionally. Turn off "Sauté" function on your Instant Pot.
- Add the chicken and pepper sauce to your Instant Pot.
- Lock the lid and ensure the valve is closed. Press the "Manual" button and cook for 7 minutes on High Pressure.
- When the cooking is done, quick release the pressure and remove the lid.
- Remove the chicken and shred using two forks.
- Return the shredded chicken and stir until well coated with the sauce.
- Serve and enjoy!

Nutrition information per serving:

- Calories: 307
- Fat: 9.6g
- Carbohydrates: 8.8g
- Dietary Fiber: 1.5g
- Protein: 45.5g

Chapter 4: Healthy Fish and Seafood Recipes

Fiery Tuna Salad with Jalapeno

Time: 10 minutes

Servings: 2

Ingredients:

- 2 (5-ounce) can of tuna,
- 8 Kalamata olives, sliced
- 1 fresh large jalapeno pepper, minced
- 2 garlic cloves, minced
- 1 tablespoon of coconut oil, melted
- 4 green or white scallions, thinly sliced
- ¼ teaspoon of organic dry mustard powder
- 1 teaspoon of crushed red pepper flakes
- 3 tablespoons of homemade Whole30-friendly mayonnaise
- 1 tablespoon of fresh parsley, chopped
- ½ teaspoon of red wine vinegar
- A pinch of organic cayenne pepper
- 1 teaspoon of sea salt (to taste)
- 1 teaspoon of freshly ground black pepper (to taste)

Instructions:

- Press the "Sauté" function on your Instant Pot and add 1 tablespoon of coconut oil.
- Once the coconut oil is melted, add the 2 minced garlic cloves and sauté until fragrant, stirring occasionally, this will take around 1 minute.
- Add the jalapeno peppers, tuna, and Kalamata olives. Cook until warmed through, stirring occasionally.
- Remove the contents to a large bowl and allow to cool.
- Stir in the scallions, dry mustard powder, crushed red pepper flakes, homemade Whole30-friendly mayonnaise, parsley, red wine vinegar, cayenne pepper, salt, and black pepper.
- Allow to chill in your refrigerator until ready to serve. Serve and enjoy!

Nutrition information per serving:

- Calories: 435
- Fat: 27.6g
- Carbohydrates: 7.8g
- Dietary Fiber: 0.8g
- Protein: 38.2g

Delicious Lemon Salmon Fillets with Garlic

Time: 12 minutes

Servings: 4

Ingredients:

- 2 pounds of frozen salmon fillets
- 2 tablespoons of olive oil, avocado oil, or coconut oil
- 2 fresh lemons, juiced
- 1 fresh lemon, thinly sliced
- 1 cup of homemade low-sodium fish stock (or water)
- A bunch of fresh herbs mix (dill, parsley, cilantro, basil, etc.)
- 2 teaspoons of garlic powder
- 1 teaspoon of sea salt (to taste)
- 1 teaspoon of freshly ground black pepper (to taste)

Instructions:

- Add the fish stock, lemon juice, and herbs to your Instant Pot. Give a good stir.
- Place a steamer rack in your Instant Pot and place the salmon fillets on top.
- Drizzle the salmon fillets with 2 tablespoons of olive oil.
- Sprinkle with garlic powder, sea salt, and freshly ground black pepper.
- Place lemon slices on top of the salmon fillets.
- Lock the lid on your Instant Pot. Press the "Manual" button and set the time to 6 minutes on High Pressure.
- When the cooking is done, quick release the pressure and remove the lid.
- Serve and enjoy!

Nutrition information per serving:

- Calories: 383
- Fat: 21.6g
- Carbohydrates: 4.1g
- Dietary Fiber: 1.2g
- Protein: 45.8g

Phenomenal Coconut Orange Salmon

Time: 25 minutes
Servings: 4
Ingredients:

- 4 (6-ounce) boneless, skinless salmon fillets
- 1 cup of unsweetened coconut milk
- 2 tablespoons of ginger, finely minced
- 2 tablespoons of coconut aminos
- 4 garlic cloves, minced
- 1 tablespoon of fish sauce
- 2 tablespoons of fresh lime juice
- 1 teaspoon of fresh orange zest
- 1 fresh medium-sized orange, juiced
- 1 fresh medium-sized orange, thinly sliced
- ¼ cup of fresh cilantro, finely chopped
- 1 teaspoon of freshly ground black pepper (to taste)

Instructions:

- Press the "Sauté" function on your Instant Pot and the orange juice, orange zest, unsweetened coconut milk, coconut aminos, garlic, ginger, fish sauce, and lime juice to your Instant Pot. Give a good stir and allow to simmer for a few minutes.
- Add the salmon and allow to simmer for 3 to 6 minutes or until the salmon is pink and opaque.
- Transfer the salmon fillets to serving plates and ladle the coconut orange sauce over the salmon.
- Top with orange slices, cilantro, and black pepper.

Nutrition information per serving:

- Calories: 416
- Fat: 25g
- Carbohydrates: 17.7g
- Dietary Fiber: 4.5g
- Protein: 35.5g

Award Winning Seafood Chili

Time: 20 minutes   Servings: 6

Ingredients:

- 1 pound of shrimp, peeled, tails removed, and deveined
- ½ pounds of scallops, cleaned
- 2 large fish steaks, cut into bite-sized pieces
- 1 pound of mussels, cleaned
- 6 ounces of clams, cleaned
- 2 tablespoons of olive oil or coconut oil
- 1 (14-ounce) can of diced tomatoes, undrained
- 3 cups of low-sodium fish stock or clam juice
- 1 large yellow onion, chopped
- 1 jalapeno pepper, finely chopped
- 1 sweet medium-sized yellow bell pepper, finely chopped
- 1 sweet medium-sized red bell pepper, finely chopped
- 1 sweet medium-sized green bell pepper, finely chopped

Spice Ingredients:

- 1 teaspoon of organic ground cumin
- ½ tablespoon of fresh oregano
- 2 teaspoons of garlic powder
- 2 teaspoons of smoked paprika
- 1 tablespoon of chili powder
- 1 teaspoon of organic ground coriander
- 1 teaspoon of sea salt (to taste)
- 1 teaspoon of freshly ground black pepper (to taste)
- A pinch of cayenne pepper
- A small pinch of organic ground cinnamon

Instructions:

- Press the "Sauté" function on your Instant Pot and add the olive oil or coconut oil.
- Once hot and ready, add the onions, red bell pepper, yellow bell pepper, green bell pepper, and jalapenos to your Instant Pot. Sauté for 3 to 5 minutes or until softened, stirring occasionally.
- Add the can of diced tomatoes, fish stock, all the spices, and bite-sized pieces of fish steaks. Stir until well combined.
- Stir in the shrimp, mussels, and clams.
- Lock the lid on your Instant Pot. Press the "Manual" button and cook for 6 minutes on High Pressure.
- When the cooking is done, naturally release the pressure for 10 minutes and quickly release the remaining pressure. Carefully remove the lid.
- Check if the mussels and clams are opened. If not, press "Sauté" and allow to simmer until opened. Adjust the seasoning as needed. Serve and enjoy!

Nutrition information per serving:

- Calories: 322
- Fat: 9.5g
- Carbohydrates: 15g
- Dietary Fiber: 1.7g
- Protein: 43.2g

Family Favorite Creole Seafood Gumbo

Time: 25 minutes

Servings: 6

Ingredients:

- 2 pounds of sea bass fillets, cut into bite-sized pieces
- 2 pounds of shrimp, peeled and deveined
- 2 sweet bell peppers, finely chopped
- 4 celery ribs, chopped
- 3 bay leaves
- 1 ½ cup of homemade low-sodium fish stock or water
- 1 (28-ounce) can of diced tomatoes
- ¼ cup of tomato paste
- 3 tablespoons of avocado oil, coconut oil, or ghee
- 2 medium-sized yellow onions, finely chopped
- ¼ cup of cilantro, freshly chopped
- 3 tablespoons of Cajun seasoning
- 1 teaspoon of sea salt (to taste)
- 1 teaspoon of freshly ground black pepper (to taste)

Instructions:

- Season the sea bass fillets with salt, black pepper, and half of the Cajun seasoning.
- Press the "Sauté" function on your Instant pot and add the oil or ghee.
- Once hot, add the fish pieces and cook for 3 minutes or until lightly browned on each side. Remove the fish pieces to a large plate and set aside.
- Add the onions, celery, bell peppers, and remaining Cajun seasoning to your Instant Pot. Sauté for 3 minutes or until softened, stirring occasionally. Turn off "Sauté" function.
- Return the cooked fish to your Instant Pot along with the tomatoes, tomato paste, bay leaves, and fish stock. Give a good stir.
- Place and seal the lid on your Instant Pot. Press the "Manual" button and set the time to 5 minutes on High Pressure.
- When the cooking is done, quick release the pressure and remove the lid
- Stir the shrimp and allow to cook until pink and opaque.
- Season with salt and black pepper. Top with fresh cilantro.
- Serve and enjoy!

Nutrition information per serving:

- Calories: 365
- Fat: 13.7g
- Carbohydrates: 12.1g
- Dietary Fiber: 3.5g
- Protein: 41g

Signature Wild Salmon with Orange-Garlic Glazed

Time: 15 minutes
Servings: 2
Ingredients:

- 2 (10-ounce) boneless, skinless salmon fillets
- 2 tablespoons of ghee, melted
- 2 garlic cloves, minced
- 2 tablespoons of rosemary
- 1 orange, zest
- 2 oranges, juice
- 1 teaspoon of sea salt (to taste)
- ½ teaspoon of freshly ground black pepper
- 1 cup of water (for your Instant Pot)

Instructions:

- Place each salmon fillets onto a large piece of parchment paper. Tightly fold the parchment paper.
- Add 1 cup of water and a steamer basket to your Instant Pot. Place the salmon packet on top of the steamer basket.
- Lock the lid on your Instant Pot. Press the "Manual" button and set the time to 3 minutes on High Pressure.
- When the cooking is done, quick release the pressure and carefully remove the lid. Remove the salmon packets and unfold the parchment paper.
- In a bowl, add 2 tablespoons of ghee, 2 minced garlic, 2 tablespoons of rosemary, orange zest, juices from 2 orange, salt, and black pepper. Mix well.
- Brush the orange-garlic glaze over the salmon fillets and place on top of the steamer basket.
- Place and seal the lid on your Instant Pot. Press the "Manual" button and cook at low pressure for 1 minute.
- When the cooking is done, quick release the pressure and remove the lid.
- Remove the salmon fillets and set to a serving plate.
- Serve and enjoy!

Nutrition information per serving:

- Calories: 617
- Fat: 30.6g
- Carbohydrates: 32.4g
- Dietary Fiber: 6.6g
- Protein: 57.6g

Gorgeous Salmon Fillets with Great-Tasting Avocado Salsa

Time: 15 minutes
Servings: 4
Ingredients:

- 4 (4-ounce) salmon fillets
- 2 teaspoons of avocado oil or coconut oil
- 1 teaspoon of sea salt (to taste)
- 1 teaspoon of freshly ground black pepper (to taste)
- 2 ripe medium-sized avocados, peeled, pitted, and chopped
  3 tablespoons of fresh cilantro, chopped
- 1 lime, juice
- 1 medium-sized sweet red bell pepper, finely chopped

Instructions:

- Season the salmon fillets with salt and black pepper.
- Press the "Sauté" function on your Instant Pot and set the temperature to the lowest setting.
- Once hot, add the salmon and cook for 4 to 5 minutes per side until cooked through. Remove and set aside. Turn off "Sauté" function.
- In a bowl, add the avocados, cilantro, lime juice, and sweet red bell pepper. Stir until well combined.
- Spoon the avocado salsa on top of the salmon fillets.
- Serve and enjoy!

Nutrition information per serving:

- Calories: 245
- Fat: 14g
- Carbohydrates: 3.85g
- Dietary Fiber: 1.9g
- Protein: 24.3g

Well-Done Coconut Lime Shrimp

Time: 30 minutes
Servings: 4
Ingredients:

- 1 pound of shrimp, peeled and deveined
- ½ onions, chopped
- 1 ¾ cups of unsweetened coconut milk
- 1 lime, juice
- 1 tablespoon of coconut aminos
- 2 garlic cloves, minced
- 1 tablespoon of coconut oil
- 1 teaspoon of fresh ginger, grated
- ¼ cup of fresh cilantro, chopped (for serving)
- 1 teaspoon of sea salt (for serving)
- 1 teaspoon of freshly ground black pepper (for serving)

Instructions:

- Press "Sauté" function on your Instant Pot and add 1 tablespoon of coconut oil, onions, and garlic cloves to your pot. Allow to sauté for 1 to 2 minutes, stirring occasionally.
- Add the 1 teaspoon of freshly grated ginger to the pot and sauté for 30 seconds.
- Stir in the coconut milk and coconut aminos to your Instant Pot.
- Add the shrimp to the coconut mixture and cook for 4 to 8 minutes or until pink and opaque.
- Add the fresh lime juice to your Instant Pot and turn off "Sauté" function.
- Serve and enjoy!

Nutrition information per serving:

- Calories: 417
- Fat: 30.4g
- Carbohydrates: 10.1g
- Dietary Fiber: 2.6g
- Protein: 28.5g

Wicked Calamari with Tomato Sauce

Time: 43 minutes

Servings: 4

Ingredients:

- 2 pounds of fresh calamari tubes and tentacles, cleaned with cold water
- 1 (14.5-ounce) can of diced tomatoes
- 1 (6-ounce) can of natural tomato paste
- 2 anchovies
- 1 teaspoon of crushed red pepper flakes
- 1 fresh lemon, juiced
- 2 tablespoon of coconut oil
- ½ cup of white wine
- 2 teaspoons of apple cider vinegar
- 1 garlic clove, minced
- 1 tablespoon of fresh parsley, chopped
- 1 teaspoon of sea salt (to taste)
- 1 teaspoon of freshly ground black pepper (to taste)

Instructions:

- Press "Sauté" function on your Instant Pot and add 2 tablespoons of coconut oil.
- Turn the "Sauté" setting to the lowest temperature.
- Once the oil is hot and ready, add the minced garlic, 2 anchovies, and 1 teaspoon of crushed red pepper flakes.
- Add the calamari and cook until lightly colored, this will take around 5 minutes.
- Add the white wine and apple cider vinegar to your Instant Pot. Allow to simmer until almost evaporated, this will take around 3 minutes.
- Stir in the diced tomatoes and tomato paste to your Instant Pot.
- Place and seal the lid on your Instant Pot. Press the "Manual" button and set the time to 19 minutes at High Pressure.
- When the cooking is done, quick release the pressure and remove the lid.
- Stir in the fresh lemon juice, fresh parsley, sea salt, and ground black pepper. Stir well.
- Serve and enjoy!

Nutrition information per serving:

- Calories: 235
- Fat: 9.2g
- Carbohydrates: 15.8g
- Dietary Fiber: 3g
- Protein: 20.7g

Scrumptious Shrimp and Mango Curry

Time: 30 minutes   Servings: 4

Ingredients:

- 2 tablespoons of coconut oil
- 1 tablespoon of ghee
- 2-inch ginger slices, finely chopped or minced
- 2 fresh green chilies, finely chopped
- 2 ½ teaspoons of organic natural Kashmiri red chili powder
- 1 small yellow onion, finely chopped
- 1 sprig of curry leaves
- 2 garlic cloves, minced
- ½ teaspoons of fenugreek seeds
- 1 teaspoon of organic mustard seeds
- 1 ½ teaspoon of organic ground coriander powder
- 1 large red tomato, finely chopped
- ¼ cup of water
- 1 medium-sized raw mango, peeled and diced
- 15 to 20 shrimp pieces, peeled and deveined
- 1 cup of unsweetened coconut milk
- ¼ teaspoon of organic ground turmeric powder
- 1 teaspoon of sea salt (to taste)
- 1 teaspoon of freshly ground black pepper (to taste)

Instructions:

- Press the "Sauté" function on your Instant Pot and add 2 tablespoons of coconut oil.
- Once the coconut oil is melted and hot, add ½ teaspoon of fenugreek seeds and 1 teaspoon of mustard seeds. Allow to sauté for a couple of seconds. Be extra attentive to not burn the seeds.
- Add 1 finely chopped yellow onions to your Instant Pot and sauté for 2 minutes, stirring occasionally.
- Add 2 minced garlic cloves, minced ginger, chopped green chiles, a sprig of curry leaves, and sea salt to your Instant Pot. Allow to sauté for 1 to 2 minutes or until translucent, stirring occasionally.
- Stir in 2 ½ teaspoons of Kashmiri red chili powder, 1 ½ teaspoon of ground coriander powder, ¼ teaspoon of ground turmeric powder, chopped tomatoes, ¼ cup of water, shrimp pieces, and mango pieces.
- Close and seal the lid on your Instant Pot. Press the "Manual" button and set the time to 10 minutes on High Pressure.
- When the cooking is completed, allow for a full natural release method and carefully remove the lid.
- Stir in the unsweetened coconut milk, ghee, and ground black pepper until well combined. Adjust the seasoning as needed. Serve and enjoy!

Nutrition information per serving:

- Calories: 502
- Fat: 51.4g
- Carbohydrates: 13.4g
- Dietary Fiber: 4.7g
- Protein: 4.7g

Delightful Fish Tacos

Time: 20 minutes
Servings: 2
Ingredients:

- 2 tilapia fillets
- 2 teaspoons of coconut oil, melted
- 1 teaspoon of sea salt (to taste)
- 2 tablespoons of smoked paprika
- 1 lime, juice
- 2 tablespoons of fresh cilantro, chopped
- 2 to 4 lettuce leaves (for taco wrap)

White Sauce Ingredients:

- ½ cup of homemade Whole30-friendly mayonnaise
- 1 tablespoon of fresh lime juice
- 1 teaspoon of dried oregano
- ½ teaspoon of organic ground cumin powder
- A pinch of cayenne pepper

Instructions:

- To make the white sauce: Add all the white sauce ingredients to a large bowl and stir with a wooden spoon until well combined.
- Place each tilapia fillets in a separate large piece of parchment paper.
- For each tilapia fillet: Drizzle with 1 teaspoon of canola oil and lime juice. Sprinkle with salt, smoked paprika, and cilantro.
- Tightly fold the parchment paper into a packet.
- Add 1 ½ cups of water and a trivet to your Instant Pot.
- Place the tilapia packet on top of the trivet.
- Place and seal the lid on your Instant Pot. Press the "Manual" button and set the time to 8 minutes on High Pressure.
- When the cooking is done, quick release the pressure and carefully remove the lid.
- Remove the tilapia packets and carefully unfold the parchment paper.
- Cut the tilapia fillets into the desired number of fish pieces.
- Place the fish on the lettuce leaves and spread the white sauce.
- Serve and enjoy!

Nutrition information per serving:

- Calories: 367
- Fat: 25.2g
- Carbohydrates: 15.9g
- Dietary Fiber: 0.1g
- Protein: 21.7g

Traditional Squid Stew

Time: 35 minutes
Servings: 4
Ingredients:

- 2 tablespoons of olive oil or natural organic ghee
- 1 pound of squid, cleaned and cut into separate rings
- 1 sweet green bell pepper, chopped
- 1 sweet red bell pepper, chopped
- 1 large yellow onion, finely chopped
- 4 garlic cloves, minced
- 2 (14.5-ounce) can of diced tomatoes, undrained
- ¼ cup of red wine
- 1 tablespoon of fresh parsley, chopped
- A pinch of crushed red pepper flakes
- 1 teaspoon of fresh thyme leaves
- 1 teaspoon of sea salt (to taste)
- 1 teaspoon of freshly ground black pepper (to taste)

Instructions:

- Press the "Sauté" function on your Instant Pot and add the olive oil.
- Once the oil is hot and ready, add the squid and cook until golden brown, stirring occasionally, this will take around 5 minutes.
- Add the chopped yellow onion and minced garlic cloves to your cooking pot and cook for an extra 2 minutes, stirring occasionally.
- Add the green bell pepper and red bell pepper to your Instant Pot and cook for an additional minute, stirring occasionally.
- Add the remaining ingredients to your Instant Pot and stir until well combined.
- Place and seal the lid on your Instant Pot. Press the "Manual" button and set the time to 20 minutes at High Pressure.
- When the cooking is done, allow for a full natural release method and carefully remove the lid.
- Press "Sauté" function again and allow to simmer for around 5 minutes.
- Serve and enjoy!

Nutrition information per serving:

- Calories: 236
- Fat: 9.2g
- Carbohydrates: 19g
- Dietary Fiber: 3.9g
- Protein: 20.4g

Flavorful Mediterranean Style Fish

Time: 20 minutes
Servings: 4
Ingredients:

- 4 white fish fillets, cleaned
- 1 tablespoon of olive oil
- 1 cup of Kalamata olives, sliced in half
- 1 pound of fresh red cherry tomatoes, sliced in half
- 2 tablespoons of pickled capers
- 1 garlic clove, minced, crushed
- 1 bunch of fresh thyme
- 1 teaspoon of sea salt (to taste)
- 1 teaspoon of freshly ground black pepper (to taste)

Instructions:

- Add 2 cups of water and a trivet inside your Instant Pot.
- In a heat-safe bowl that fits inside your Instant Pot, add the cherry tomatoes and fresh thyme.
- Place the 4 white fish fillets on top of the cherry tomatoes.
- Add the garlic, olive oil, salt, and black pepper over the fish fillets.
- Place the heat-safe bowl on top of the trivet in your Instant Pot.
- Place and seal the lid on your Instant Pot. Press the "Manual" button and cook for 5 minutes at High Pressure.
- When the cooking is done, naturally release the pressure and carefully remove the lid.
- Remove the bowl and divide into serving plates.
- Top with olives and capers.
- Serve and enjoy!

Nutrition information per serving:

- Calories: 301
- Fat: 18.5g
- Carbohydrates: 22g
- Dietary Fiber: 2.9g
- Protein: 14.6g

Perfectly Steamed Mussels

Time: 15 minutes
Servings: 12
Ingredients:

- 5 pounds of fresh and raw mussel, rinsed and cleaned
- 1 cup of white cooking wine
- 6 tablespoons of cashew butter, almond butter, or ghee
- 4 medium-sized yellow onions, finely chopped
- 4 garlic cloves, minced
- 1 ½ cup of homemade low-sodium chicken broth
- ¼ cup of fresh parsley leaves, finely chopped
- 3 fresh lemons, squeezed
- 1 teaspoon of sea salt (to taste)

Instructions:

- Press the "Sauté" function on your Instant Pot and add the nut butter or ghee.
- Once melted, add the onions and cook for approximately 2 minutes or until lightly brown, stirring occasionally.
- Add the garlic and sauté for 1 minute or until translucent, stirring occasionally.
- Deglaze your Instant Pot with the 1 cup of white cooking wine. Allow to cook for a couple of minutes until some of the cooking wine evaporates and the sauce thickens, stirring occasionally.
- Stir in the fresh parsley leaves to your Instant Pot.
- Add the fresh mussels, chicken broth, and juices from the lemon to your Instant Pot.
- Lock the lid on your Instant Pot. Press the "Manual" button and set the time to 3 minutes on High Pressure.
- When the cooking is done, quick release the pressure and carefully remove the lid.
- Transfer the mussels to a large bowl and sprinkle with sea salt.
- Serve and enjoy!

Nutrition information per serving:

- Calories: 255
- Fat: 10.3g
- Carbohydrates: 12.8g
- Dietary Fiber: 1.3g
- Protein: 23.8g

Oozing Buttery Lobster Tails

Time: 13 minutes
Servings: 2
Ingredients:

- 2 frozen lobster tails
- 1 cup of homemade low-sodium fish stock (or water will be fine)
- 1 teaspoon of celery salt
- 1 teaspoon of black pepper
- A pinch of organic cayenne pepper
- A pinch of organic ground cinnamon

Yummy Cashew Butter Sauce Ingredients:

- 1 cup of cashew butter
- 2 garlic cloves, minced
- 1 teaspoon of sea salt
- ½ teaspoon of freshly ground black pepper
- 2 teaspoons of fresh lemon juice
- 1 teaspoon of fresh dill, chopped

Instructions:

- Using kitchen shears or a sharp knife, carefully make an incision down the middle of each lobster tail until the lobster flesh is exposed.
- Add the fish stock, celery salt, black pepper, cayenne pepper, and cinnamon to your Instant Pot.
- Add the trivet in the bottom of the cooking pot and place the lobster tails on top.
- Place and seal the lid on your Instant Pot. Press the "Manual" button and set the time to 4 minutes on High Pressure.
- When the cooking is done, quick release the pressure and remove the lid. Place the lobster tails aside.
- To make the cashew butter sauce: In a small bowl, add all the cashew butter ingredients and microwave until the cashew butter is melted. Give a good stir.
- Place the lobster tails onto serving plates and drizzle with the cashew butter sauce.
- Serve and enjoy!

Nutrition information per serving:

- Calories: 943
- Fat: 93.3g
- Carbohydrates: 0.1g
- Dietary Fiber: 0g
- Protein: 28.5g

Chapter 5: Mouth-watering Goat and Lamb Recipes

Desirable Coconut Lime Lamb

Time: 19 minutes
Servings: 4

- 1 ½ pounds of fresh boneless lamb shoulder, trimmed and cut into bite-sized pieces
- 1 tablespoon of coconut oil or olive oil
- 1 medium-sized red onion, finely chopped
- 1 fresh red chili, finely chopped
- 1 cup of homemade low-sodium chicken stock
- 2 tablespoons of fresh lime juice
- ½ to 1 cup of unsweetened coconut cream
- 1 tablespoon of low-carb organic coconut flour
- 1 teaspoon of organic turmeric powder
- ½ teaspoon of crushed red chili flakes
- 1 teaspoon of sea salt (to taste)
- 1 teaspoon of freshly ground black pepper (to taste)

Instructions:

- Press the "Sauté" function on your Instant Pot and add the oil.
- Once the oil is hot and ready, add the lamb pieces and sauté until brown on all sides. Remove and set aside.
- Add the onions and garlic to your Instant Pot. Sauté until onions are translucent, stirring occasionally.
- Return the lamb pieces to your Instant Pot. Add the remaining ingredients except for the coconut cream and flour. Give a good stir.
- Lock the lid and ensure the valve is closed. Press the "Manual" button and cook for 8 minutes on High Pressure.
- When the cooking is done, allow for a full natural release method and naturally release the pressure. Carefully remove the lid.
- Stir in the unsweetened coconut cream and sprinkle with coconut flour. Allow to cook until thick and creamy.
- Serve and enjoy!

Nutrition information per serving:

- Calories: 417
- Fat: 23g
- Carbohydrates: 1.8g
- Dietary Fiber: 0.7g
- Protein: 48.3g

Extraordinary Sesame Garlic Lamb

Time: 33 minutes

Servings: 4

Ingredients:

* 2 pounds of boneless lamb, cut into bite-sized pieces
* ¼ cup of low-sodium coconut aminos
* 4 garlic cloves, minced
* 1 1-inch fresh ginger, finely grated
* ½ cup of homemade low-sodium chicken broth
* 2 tablespoons of sesame oil
* ¼ teaspoon of organic crushed red pepper flakes
* 2 tablespoons of almond flour
* 1 teaspoon of sea salt (to taste)
* 1 teaspoon of freshly ground black pepper (to taste)
* 2 fresh green onions, thinly sliced
* Toasted sesame seeds

Instructions:

* Add the lamb pieces, coconut aminos, sesame oil, finely grated ginger, garlic, chicken broth, salt, black pepper, and crushed red pepper flakes. Give a good stir.
* Lock the lid and ensure the valve is closed. Press the "Manual" button and cook for 5 minutes on High Pressure.
* When the cooking is done, naturally release the pressure for 10 minutes, then quick release the remaining pressure. Carefully remove the lid.
* Press the "Sauté" function to the lowest temperature by pressing the "Less" button.
* Sprinkle almond flour over the lamb pieces.
* Allow to simmer for around 5 minutes or until thickened, stirring occasionally.
* Transfer the sesame garlic lamb to serving plates and top with sesame seeds and green onions.
* Serve and enjoy!

Nutrition information per serving:

* Calories: 499
* Fat: 24g
* Carbohydrates: 2.3g
* Dietary Fiber: 0.1g
* Protein: 63.9g

Intriguing Mediterranean Goat Roast with Sweet Potato and Vegetables

Time: 1 hour

Servings: 10

Ingredients:

- 1 (5 to 6-pound) boneless or bone-in goat leg
- 2 medium-sized sweet potatoes, cut into 2-inch pieces
- 2 medium-sized sweet red bell peppers, finely chopped
- 1 small butternut squash, cut into bite-sized pieces
- 2 tablespoons of balsamic vinegar
- 2 tablespoons of coconut oil, melted
- 1 medium-sized red onion, sliced
- 4 garlic cloves, minced
- 2 tablespoons of almond flour
- 2 cups of homemade low-sodium chicken stock
- 1 teaspoon of organic sweet marjoram powder
- 2 tablespoons of fresh rosemary, finely chopped
- 1 tablespoon of fresh thyme, finely chopped
- 1 teaspoon of sea salt (to taste)
- 1 teaspoon of freshly ground black pepper (to taste)

Instructions:

- Press the "Sauté" function on your Instant Pot and add the coconut oil.
- Once the display reads hot, add the goat leg and sear until brown on both sides. Remove and set aside.
- Add the sweet potatoes, bell pepper, butternut squash, red onion, and garlic to your Instant Pot. Sauté until softened, stirring occasionally.
- Pour chicken stock into your Instant Pot. Stir in the balsamic vinegar, marjoram powder, rosemary, thyme, salt, and black pepper.
- Place the browned goat leg on top of the vegetables.
- Lock the lid and ensure the valve is closed. Press the "Manual" button and cook for 45 minutes on High Pressure.
- When the cooking is done, quick release the pressure and carefully remove the lid.
- Remove the goat leg and transfer the vegetables to a serving platter.
- Press the "Sauté" function on your Instant Pot and sprinkle with almond flour. Sauté until the liquid becomes thick, stirring occasionally.
- Spoon the gravy over the goat leg and vegetables.
- Serve and enjoy!

Nutrition information per serving:

- Calories: 585
- Fat: 23g
- Carbohydrates: 12.9g
- Dietary Fiber: 2.1g
- Protein: 64.3g

Summer Jamaican-Inspired Goat Curry

Time: 20 minutes
Servings: 6
Ingredients:

- 3 ½ pounds of fresh boneless goat meat, cut into bite-sized pieces
- 3 medium-sized sweet potatoes, peeled and cut into chunks
- ¼ cup of ghee
- 5 garlic cloves, minced
- 1 medium-sized red onion, finely chopped
- 5 tablespoons of organic curry powder
- 1 tablespoon of fresh thyme, finely chopped
- 1 tablespoon of smoked paprika
- 2 teaspoons of garam masala
- 2 tablespoons of fresh ginger, finely grated
- 1 (14.5-ounce) can of tomato sauce
- 1 cup of unsweetened coconut cream
- 1 teaspoon of sea salt (to taste)
- 1 teaspoon of white pepper (to taste)
- Fresh chopped cilantro (for serving)
- Cauliflower rice (for serving)

Instructions:

- Press the "Sauté" function on your Instant Pot and add 2 tablespoons of ghee.
- Once hot, add the onions, garlic, and ginger to your Instant Pot. Sauté for 2 minutes or until lightly browned, stirring occasionally.
- Add the goat meat and remaining ghee to your cooking pot and sauté until brown on all sides.
- Add the sweet potatoes, curry powder, thyme, smoked paprika, garam masala, tomato sauce, salt, and white pepper to your Instant Pot.
- Lock the lid and ensure the valve is closed. Press the "Manual" button and cook for 7 minutes on High Pressure.
- When the cooking is done, quick release the pressure and carefully remove the lid.
- Stir in the unsweetened coconut cream.
- Press the "Sauté" function on your Instant Pot and allow to simmer for 2 minutes or until thickened.
- Sprinkle with fresh cilantro and serve with cauliflower rice.
- Serve and enjoy!

Nutrition information per serving:

- Calories: 329
- Fat: 12g
- Carbohydrates: 12g
- Dietary Fiber: 3g
- Protein: 46g

Heavenly Cream of Mushroom Lamb with Cauliflower Risotto

Time: 35 minutes   Servings: 6

Chicken Ingredients:

- 1 ½ pounds of boneless lamb, cut into bite-sized pieces
- 1 tablespoon of coconut oil
- 1 cup of leeks, sliced
- 4 bacon slices, chopped
- 1 ½ cup of Portobello mushrooms, sliced
- 1 cup of unsweetened coconut cream
- 1 tablespoon of Dijon mustard
- 1 teaspoon of sea salt (to taste)
- 1 teaspoon of freshly ground black pepper (to taste)

Risotto Ingredients:

- 1 large head of fresh cauliflower, chopped
- 2 tablespoons of olive oil
- 3 garlic cloves, minced
- 1 small white onion, finely chopped
- 1 cup of Portobello mushrooms, sliced
- 1/3 cup of homemade low-sodium chicken stock
- 1 tablespoon of dried basil
- 3 tablespoons of fresh thyme

Instructions:

- In a food processor, add the cauliflower and pulse until rice consistency. Set aside.
- Press the "Sauté" function on your Instant Pot.
- Once hot, add the bacon and cook for 4 minutes per side or until brown and crispy. Remove and set aside. Reserve the bacon fat.
- Add the lamb pieces to your Instant Pot and cook until brown, stirring occasionally. Remove and set aside.
- Add the coconut oil, leeks and mushrooms to your Instant Pot. Sauté for 4 minutes or until softened, stirring occasionally.
- Return the bacon and lamb pieces to your Instant Pot. Stir in the coconut cream, Dijon mustard, salt, and black pepper.
- Lock the lid on your Instant Pot and ensure the valve is closed. Press the "Manual" button and cook for 8 minutes on High Pressure.
- When the cooking is done, naturally release the pressure for 5 minutes, and then quick release the remaining pressure. Carefully remove the lid.
- To make the cauliflower risotto: Heat 2 tablespoons of olive oil in a saucepan over medium-high heat. Add the garlic, onion, and mushrooms. Sauté for 4 minutes or until softened, stirring occasionally.
- Stir in the cauliflower rice, chicken stock, dried basil, and fresh thyme. Allow to simmer for a few minutes.
- Lay out the cauliflower risotto onto plates and top with the lamb pieces. Serve!

Nutrition information per serving:
Calories: 490, Fat: 30.4g, Carbohydrates: 15g, Dietary Fiber: 5.2g, Protein: 41.7g

The Number One Roman-Inspired Lamb

Time: 1 hour

Servings: 8

Ingredients:

- 3 ½ pounds of boneless fresh lamb shoulder, trimmed and cut into 2 separate pieces
- 6 fresh sprigs of thyme
- 4 fresh sprigs of rosemary
- 1 tablespoon of fresh tarragon, finely chopped
- 1 tablespoon of fresh oregano, finely chopped
- 2 tablespoons of olive oil
- 1 large red onion, finely chopped
- 1 cup of dry white wine
- 1 tablespoon of fresh lemon juice
- A pinch of organic crushed red pepper flakes
- 2 tablespoons of garlic powder or 9 minced garlic cloves
- 2 teaspoons of sea salt (to taste)
- 1 teaspoon of freshly ground black pepper (to taste)

Instructions:

- Season the lamb shoulder with garlic powder, crushed red pepper flakes, salt, thyme sprigs, rosemary sprigs, and black pepper. Refrigerate overnight.
- Press the "Sauté" function on your Instant Pot and add the olive oil.
- Once hot, add the lamb pieces and sauté for 5 to 7 minutes per side or until brown. Remove and set aside.
- Add the onion and sauté for 3 minutes or until translucent, stirring occasionally.
- Deglaze your Instant Pot with the dry white wine and allow to simmer until half of the liquid evaporates.
- Return the lamb to your Instant Pot.
- Lock the lid and ensure the valve is closed. Press the "Manual" button and cook for 50 minutes on High Pressure.
- When the cooking is done, naturally release the pressure and carefully remove the lid.
- Transfer the lamb to a serving platter.
- Press the "Sauté" function on your Instant Pot and stir in the fresh lemon juice, chopped tarragon, chopped oregano. Turn off the "Sauté" function on your Instant Pot
- Ladle the liquid over the lamb. Serve and enjoy!

Nutrition information per serving:

- Calories: 405
- Fat: 18.1g
- Carbohydrates: 1.3g
- Dietary Fiber: 0.3g
- Protein: 55.9g

Rich Lamb Chops with Rosemary and Garlic

Time: 35 minutes
Servings: 4
Ingredients:

- 2 pounds of thick lamb chops
- 4 garlic cloves, minced
- 1 tablespoon of fresh rosemary, finely chopped
- 1 fresh medium-sized lemon, zest
- ¼ cup of olive oil + 1 teaspoon of olive oil
- 1 teaspoon of onion powder
- 1 teaspoon of sea salt (to taste)
- 1 teaspoon of freshly ground black pepper (to taste)
- 1 cup of plain water

Instructions:

- In a bowl, add the garlic cloves, rosemary, lemon zest, ¼ cup of olive oil, onion powder, salt, and black pepper. Stir until well combined.
- Pour the garlic-rosemary mixture over the lamb chops and allow to marinate overnight.
- Press the "Sauté" function on your Instant Pot and add 1 teaspoon of olive oil.
- Once the display reads hot, working in batches if necessary, add the lamb chops and sauté for 4 minutes per side. Remove and set aside. Turn off "Sauté" function.
- Add 1 cup of water and a trivet to your Instant Pot.
- Place the lamb chops on top of the trivet.
- Lock the lid and ensure the valve is sealed. Press the "Manual" button and cook for 10 minutes on High Pressure.
- When the cooking is done, quick release the pressure and carefully remove the lid.
- Remove the lamb chops and allow to cool.
- Serve and enjoy!

Nutrition information per serving:

- Calories: 534
- Fat: 29.2g
- Carbohydrates: 1g
- Dietary Fiber: 0.1g
- Protein: 63.9g

Overpowering Pressure-Cooked Balsamic Rosemary Lamb Chops

Time: 35 minutes
Servings: 4
Ingredients:

- 4 thick lamb chops
- ½ cup of balsamic vinegar
- 3 sprigs of fresh rosemary
- 2 tablespoons of olive oil
- 4 garlic cloves, minced
- 1 cup of water
- 2 teaspoons of sea salt (to taste)
- 1 teaspoon of freshly ground black pepper (to taste)

Instructions:

- Press the "Sauté" function on your Instant Pot and add the olive oil.
- Once hot, add the lamb chops and sear on both sides until 4 minutes or until brown. Remove and set aside. Turn off "Sauté" function.
- Add 1 cup of water and a trivet to your Instant Pot.
- Place the lamb chops on top of the trivet.
- Close and seal the lid on your Instant Pot. Press the "Manual" button and cook for 10 minutes on High Pressure.
- When the cooking is done, quick release the pressure and carefully remove the lid.
- Remove the lamb chops and remove the trivet. Discard the water.
- Press the "Sauté" function on your Instant Pot and add 1 tablespoon of olive oil.
- Once hot, add the garlic and onions. Sauté until browned, stirring occasionally.
- Stir in the balsamic vinegar and rosemary. Allow to simmer until thick, stirring occasionally.
- Return the lamb chops to your Instant Pot and spoon the balsamic sauce over the lamb chops.
- Serve and enjoy!

Nutrition information per serving:

- Calories: 675
- Fat: 31g
- Carbohydrates: 0.3g
- Dietary Fiber: 0g
- Protein: 91.8g

Notable Greek-Inspired Lamb and Cabbage Bowls

Time:
Servings:
Ingredients:

- 1 pound of grass-fed extra lean ground lamb
- 1 cup of homemade low-sodium beef broth or chicken stock
- ½ large fresh head green cabbage, cored and shredded
- 2 tablespoons of dried cranberries
- 1 small yellow onion, finely chopped
- 2 garlic cloves, minced
- 1 tablespoon of olive oil
- ¼ cup of fresh organic tomato paste
- 1 teaspoon of smoked paprika or regular paprika
- 1 teaspoon of fresh oregano, finely chopped
- 1 teaspoon of fresh tarragon, finely chopped
- 1 teaspoon of organic ground cinnamon powder

Instructions:

- Press the "Sauté" function on your Instant Pot and add the olive oil.
- Once hot, add the onion and garlic cloves. Sauté until lightly browned, stirring occasionally.
- Add the ground lamb and cook for 4 to 6 minutes or until browned.
- Stir in the remaining ingredients until well combined.
- Lock the lid and ensure the valve is closed.
- Press the "Manual" button and cook for 15 minutes on High Pressure.
- When the cooking is done, quick release the pressure and carefully remove the lid.
- Give a good stir and adjust the seasoning as needed.
- Serve and enjoy!

Nutrition information per serving:

- Calories: 323
- Fat: 8.3g
- Carbohydrates: 35g
- Dietary Fiber: 7.8g
- Protein: 31.1g

Awesome Mango-Flavored Lamb Served with Cauliflower-Coconut Rice

Time: 21 minutes
Servings: 4
Ingredients:

- 2 pounds of fresh boneless lamb shoulder, well-trimmed and cut into 2-inch pieces
- 2 tablespoons of coconut oil
- A small pinch of organic cayenne pepper
- A small pinch of organic ground cinnamon powder
- 1 teaspoon of sea salt (to taste)
- 1 teaspoon of freshly ground black pepper (to taste)
- 1 cup of homemade fresh mango juice
- ½ cup of homemade low-sodium organic chicken stock
- 1 1-inch piece of ginger, peeled and finely grated
- 1 tablespoon of low-sodium coconut aminos
- 1 teaspoon of coconut flour
- 1 teaspoon of minced garlic
- ½ teaspoon of fresh Habanero pepper, finely chopped
- Fresh mango cubes (for serving)

Cauliflower-Coconut Rice Ingredients:

- 4 cups of cauliflower, chopped into florets
- 4 tablespoons of unsweetened grated coconut flakes
- 1 tablespoon of coconut oil
- A small pinch of organic sea salt

Instructions:

- Season the lamb pieces with cayenne pepper, cinnamon powder, salt, and freshly ground black pepper
- Press the "Sauté" function on your Instant Pot and add 1 tablespoon of olive to your Instant Pot.
- Once the display reads hot, working in batches if necessary, add the lamb pieces and cook until brown on all sides. Remove and set aside.
- Add the remaining tablespoon of coconut oil to your Instant Pot.
- Once hot, add the ginger, garlic, and Habanero pepper to your Instant Pot. Sauté until fragrant, stirring occasionally.
- Stir in the mango, mango juice, chicken stock, coconut aminos, and lime juice to your Instant Pot. Sprinkle the 1 teaspoon of coconut flour over.
- Lock the lid and ensure the valve is closed. Press the "Manual" button and cook for 8 minutes on High Pressure.

- When the cooking is done, naturally release the pressure for 10 minutes, and then quick release the remaining pressure. Carefully remove the lid.
- In a food processor, add the cauliflower florets and process until rice-like consistency.
- In a large skillet, add 1 tablespoon of coconut oil over medium-high heat and add cauliflower rice and unsweetened grated coconut flakes. Cook for 3 minutes or until tender, stirring occasionally. Alternatively, you can prepare the cauliflower-coconut rice in a second Instant Pot using the "Sauté" function.
- Transfer the mango-marinated lamb and mango cubes into bowls of cauliflower coconut rice.
- Serve and enjoy!

Nutrition information per serving:

- Calories: 632
- Fat: 32g
- Carbohydrates: 39.3gg
- Dietary Fiber: 5.83g
- Protein: 31.3g

Deluxe Moroccan-Inspired Goat Stew

Time: 30 minutes   Servings: 6

Ingredients:

- 1 pound of fresh boneless goat meat, cut into bite-sized pieces
- 2 tablespoons of olive oil or ghee
- 4 medium-sized orange carrots, chopped
- 1 medium-sized red onion, finely chopped
- 2 (14.5-ounce) cans of crushed tomatoes, undrained
- 4 garlic cloves, minced
- 1 medium-sized sweet potatoes, peeled and chopped into chunks
- 3 unsweetened dried apricots, cut into small pieces
- 4 cups of kale, stemmed and roughly chopped
- 3 cups of homemade low-sodium organic chicken stock
- 3 tablespoons of low-sodium coconut aminos
- 1 teaspoon of organic ground cinnamon powder
- ½ teaspoon of organic ground curry powder
- 1 teaspoon of smoked paprika
- ½ teaspoon of organic ground turmeric powder
- 1 teaspoon of organic ground ginger powder
- A small pinch of cayenne pepper
- 1 teaspoon of sea salt (to taste)
- 1 teaspoon of freshly ground black pepper (to taste)

Instructions:

- Press the "Sauté" function on your Instant Pot and add 1 tablespoon of olive oil.
- Once the display reads hot, add the goat pieces and sauté for 4 minutes or until brown, stirring occasionally. Remove and set aside.
- Add the remaining tablespoon of olive oil.
- Once hot, add the minced garlic and finely chopped red onions. Sauté for 3 minutes or until lightly browned, stirring occasionally.
- Return the goat meat and the rest of the goat stew ingredients to your Instant Pot. Give a good stir.
- Lock the lid and ensure the valve is closed. Press the "Manual" button and cook for 20 minutes on High Pressure.
- When the cooking is done, naturally release the pressure and carefully remove the lid.
- Stir the stew again and adjust the seasoning as needed. Serve and enjoy!

Nutrition information per serving:

- Calories: 267
- Fat: 10.8g
- Carbohydrates: 18.5g
- Dietary Fiber: 4g
- Protein: 24.9g

Unique Sweet and Sour Lamb

Time: 20 minutes   Servings: 4

Lamb Ingredients:

- 1 ½ pounds of boneless fresh lamb shoulder, cut into 2-inch pieces
- 2 fresh medium-sized sweet green peppers, finely chopped
- 1 fresh medium-sized sweet red bell pepper finely chopped
- 1 medium-sized red onion, finely chopped
- 2 tablespoons of coconut oil, olive oil, or ghee
- 2 teaspoons of fresh ginger, minced
- 1 ½ cup of fresh pineapple chunks
- 1 cup of organic homemade low-sodium chicken stock
- 1 teaspoon of sea salt (to taste)
- 1 teaspoon of freshly ground black pepper (to taste)

Sweet and Sour Sauce Ingredients:

- ½ cup of fresh pineapple juice (Not store-bought, it must be fresh)
- 1/3 cup of homemade sugar-free tomato ketchup
- ¼ cup of low sodium coconut aminos
- ¼ cup of organic rice vinegar
- 1 tablespoon of coconut flour

Instructions:

- Season the lamb pieces with salt and black pepper
- Press the "Sauté" function on your Instant Pot and add 1 tablespoon of coconut oil.
- Once hot, add the lamb pieces and cook until brown, stirring occasionally. Remove and set aside.
- Add the remaining tablespoon of coconut oil to your Instant Pot. Once hot, red onions, ginger, and bell peppers to your Instant Pot. Sauté for 2 minutes, stirring occasionally.
- Turn off "Sauté" function on your Instant Pot. Return the lamb pieces and add the pineapple chunks and chicken stock to your Instant Pot.
- Close and seal the lid on your Instant Pot. Press the "Manual" button and cook for 10 minutes on High Pressure.
- When the cooking is done, naturally release the pressure and carefully remove the lid.
- In a bowl, add and mix ½ cup of fresh pineapple juice, 1/3 cup of sugar-free ketchup, ¼ cup of coconut aminos, and ¼ cup of rice vinegar. Mix well.
- Press the "Sauté" function on your Instant Pot and pour the sweet and sour sauce over the lamb pieces. Sprinkle 1 tablespoon of coconut flour and cook until thick.
- Serve and enjoy!

Nutrition information per serving:

- Calories: 464
- Fat: 19.7g
- Carbohydrates: 22.6g
- Dietary Fiber: 2.4g
- Protein: 49.3g

Terrific Barbecue Lamb Meatloaf

Time: 30 minutes

Servings: 4

Ingredients:

- 1 pound of lean ground lamb
- 6 bacon slices, cooked and minced
- ½ medium-sized red onion, finely grated
- 2 garlic cloves, minced
- ¼ cup of cilantro, finely chopped
- ¼ cup of coconut or almond flour
- 2 tablespoons of Whole30-friendly homemade barbecue sauce
- 1 teaspoon of liquid smoke
- 1 large egg, beaten
- 1 teaspoon of sea salt (to taste)
- 1 teaspoon of freshly ground black pepper (to taste)

Instructions:

- Add 1 cup of water and a trivet to your Instant Pot.
- In a large bowl, add the ground lamb, grated red onion, minced garlic cloves, flour, cilantro, liquid smoke, large egg, salt, and black pepper. Stir until well combined.
- Form the ground lamb mixture into a meatloaf shape.
- Spread the barbecue sauce over the meatloaf.
- Wrap and fold the aluminum foil around the meatloaf. Place the meatloaf on top of the trivet.
- Close and seal the lid on your Instant Pot. Press the "Manual" button and cook for 20 minutes on High Pressure.
- When the cooking is done, naturally release the pressure and carefully remove the lid.
- Remove the meatloaf from your Instant Pot and allow to cool.
- Serve and enjoy!

Nutrition information per serving:

- Calories: 409
- Fat: 22.2g
- Carbohydrates: 5g
- Dietary Fiber: 0.5g
- Protein: 44.3g

Godly Irish-Inspired Lamb Stew

Time: 1 hour and 30 minutes
Servings: 6
Ingredients:

- 1 pound of boneless lamb shoulder, cut into bite-sized pieces
- 1 pound of yellow potatoes, chopped into chunks
- 2 tablespoons of coconut flour
- 2 tablespoons of olive oil
- 2 bay leaves
- 4 cups of homemade low-sodium organic chicken stock
- 1 medium-sized red onion, finely chopped
- 1 fresh sprig of rosemary
- 1 fresh sprig of thyme
- 1 ½ cup of fresh orange carrots, thickly sliced
- 1 cup of Portobello mushrooms, sliced
- 4 bacon slices, finely chopped
- 1 teaspoon of sea salt
- 1 teaspoon of freshly ground black pepper

Instructions:

- Season the lamb pieces with salt and black pepper. Coat with 2 tablespoons of coconut flour.
- Press the "Sauté" function on your Instant Pot and add the olive oil.
- Once hot, add the lamb pieces and bacon bits. Sauté until brown on all sides, stirring occasionally.
- Add the remaining ingredients to your Instant Pot.
- Close and seal the lid on your Instant Pot. Press the "Manual" button and cook for 10 minutes on High Pressure.
- When the cooking is done, naturally release the pressure for 10 minutes, then quick release the remaining pressure. Carefully remove the lid.
- Stir the stew again and adjust the seasoning as needed.
- Serve and enjoy!

Nutrition information per serving:

- Calories: 268
- Fat: 13g
- Carbohydrates: 19.3g
- Dietary Fiber: 2.9g
- Protein: 23g

Marvelous Lamb Meatballs with Tomato Sauce

Time: 25 minutes

Servings: 6

Ingredients:

- 2 pounds of lean ground lamb
- 1 medium-sized red onion, peeled and finely chopped
- 3 tablespoons of olive oil
- ¼ cup of unsweetened coconut cream
- 2 large eggs
- 3 garlic cloves, minced
- ¼ cup of coconut flour
- ½ teaspoon of crushed red pepper flakes
- ½ teaspoon of organic cayenne pepper powder
- 1 teaspoon of organic ground cinnamon powder
- ¼ cup of fresh parsley leaves, finely chopped
- 1 teaspoon of sea salt (to taste)
- 1 teaspoon of freshly ground black pepper (to taste)
- 1 tablespoon of dried oregano
- 1 (28-ounce) can of crushed tomatoes
- 1 (14.5-ounce) can of tomato sauce

Instructions:

- In a large bowl, add the ground lamb, red onion, coconut cream, eggs, garlic, coconut flour, crushed red pepper flakes, cayenne pepper powder, cinnamon powder, parsley, salt, black pepper, and oregano. Stir until well incorporated together.
- Form the lamb mixture into meatballs.
- Press the "Sauté" function on your Instant Pot and add the 3 tablespoons of olive oil.
- Working in batches, add the meatballs and sauté until brown on all sides. Repeat until all the meatballs are brown. Turn off "Sauté" setting.
- Add all the meatballs to your Instant Pot and pour the crushed tomatoes and tomato sauce over the meatballs.
- Lock the lid and ensure the valve is closed. Press the "Manual" button and cook for 7 minutes on High Pressure.
- When the cooking is done, naturally release the pressure for 5 minutes, and then quick release the remaining pressure. Carefully remove the lid.
- Give the meatballs a gentle stir until well coated with the sauce. Adjust the seasoning if necessary.
- Serve and enjoy!

Nutrition information per serving:

- Calories: 463
- Fat: 23.3g
- Carbohydrates: 15.7g
- Dietary Fiber: 6.7g
- Protein: 47.6g

Chapter 6: Delicious Beef and Pork Recipes

The Best Pork Carnitas

Time: 33 minutes

Servings: 6

Ingredients:

- 2 pounds of fresh boneless pork tenderloin, well-trimmed and cut into large pieces
- 4 garlic cloves, crushed
- 2 tablespoons of olive oil, coconut oil, or avocado oil
- 1 tablespoon of dried oregano
- 1 tablespoon of fresh parsley, finely chopped
- 1 teaspoon of smoked paprika
- 2 teaspoons of organic ground cumin powder
- 1 teaspoon of chili powder
- 1 teaspoon of sea salt (to taste)
- 1 teaspoon of freshly ground black pepper (to taste)
- 1 teaspoon of organic ground cinnamon powder
- ¾ cup of fresh orange juice
- ¼ cup of fresh pineapple juice
- 1/3 cup of fresh lime juice

Instructions:

- In a bowl, add all the ingredients except for the pork and olive oil.
- Press the "Sauté" function on your Instant Pot and add the olive oil.
- Once hot, add the pork pieces and sear for 4 minutes per side or until brown. Turn off "Sauté" function on your Instant Pot.
- Add the liquid combination to your Instant Pot.
- Lock the lid and ensure the valve is closed. Press the "Manual" button and cook for 15 minutes on High Pressure. When the cooking is done, quick release the pressure and carefully remove the lid.
- Transfer the pork pieces to a serving platter and shred using two forks.
- Line a baking sheet lined with parchment paper. Broil inside your broiler for 4 minutes. Be careful not to burn the pork.
- Serve and enjoy!

Nutrition information per serving:

- Calories: 279
- Fat: 10.1g
- Carbohydrates: 5.2g
- Dietary Fiber: 0.1g
- Protein: 40g

Amazingly Delicious Korean Beef

Time: 23 minutes
Servings: 6
Ingredients:

- 3 pounds of fresh boneless flank steak, cut into bite-sized pieces
- ½ cup of homemade low-sodium organic beef stock
- 1/3 cup of low-sodium coconut aminos
- 4 garlic cloves, minced
- 1 teaspoon of Sriracha sauce (to taste)
- ½ teaspoon of onion powder
- 1 teaspoon of sea salt (to taste)
- ½ teaspoon of freshly ground black pepper (to taste)
- 1 tablespoon of sesame oil
- 1 1-inch fresh ginger, peeled and finely grated
- 1 tablespoon of rice wine vinegar
- 3 tablespoons of almond flour
- 2 green onions, thinly sliced (for serving)
- 1 tablespoon of toasted seem seeds (for serving)

Instructions:

- In a bowl, add and mix all the ingredients except for the almond flour and flank steak.
- Add the flank steak pieces to your Instant Pot and stir in the beef broth mixture.
- Lock the lid and ensure the valve is closed. Press the "Manual" button and cook for 15 minutes on High Pressure.
- When the cooking is done, manually release the pressure and carefully remove the lid.
- Press the "Sauté" function on your Instant Pot and stir in the almond flour. Allow to cook until thickens, this will take around 3 minutes, stirring occasionally.
- Garnish with green onions slices and toasted sesame seeds.
- Serve and enjoy!

Nutrition information per serving:

- Calories: 540
- Fat: 18.4g
- Carbohydrates: 4.1g
- Dietary Fiber: 1.7g
- Protein: 86g

Party-Perfect Steak Fajitas

Time: 13 minutes
Servings: 8
Ingredients:

- 1 pound of organic flank steak, sliced into thin strips
- 1 tablespoon of organic taco seasoning
- 1 teaspoon of regular or smoked paprika
- 1 medium-sized green bell peppers, sliced
- 1 medium-sized red bell pepper, sliced
- 1 medium-sized red onions, thinly sliced
- 1 (14.5-ounce) can of diced tomatoes with green chiles, undrained
- ¼ cup of organic homemade low-sodium beef broth
- ¼ cup of fresh cilantro, finely chopped
- 1 tablespoon of lime juice
- 1 teaspoon of lime zest
- A small pinch of crushed red pepper flakes
- 1 teaspoon of sea salt (to taste)
- 1 teaspoon of freshly ground black pepper (to taste)

Instructions:

- Add all the ingredients to your Instant Pot and give a good stir.
- Lock the lid and ensure the valve is closed. Press the "Manual" button and cook for 8 minutes on High Pressure.
- When the cooking is done, naturally release the pressure and carefully remove the lid.
- Give a good stir and adjust the seasoning if necessary.
- Serve and enjoy over cauliflower rice.

Nutrition information per serving:

- Calories: 164
- Fat: 4.3g
- Carbohydrates: 8.7g
- Dietary Fiber: 3.2g
- Protein: 15.3g

Fashionable Pork Steaks with Cremini Mushrooms, Sweet Potatoes, and Gravy

Time: 33 minutes   Servings: 6

Ingredients:

- 2 ½ pounds of organic pork shoulder steaks trimmed
- ½ pounds of Cremini mushrooms, sliced or chopped
- 4 medium-sized sweet potatoes, chopped
- ¼ cup of unsweetened coconut cream
- 2 tablespoons of almond or coconut flour
- 2 tablespoons of organic Dijon mustard (if store-bought make sure you check ingredients for any unfriendly Whole30 ingredients)
- 2 tablespoons of fresh lime juice
- 1 tablespoon of dried oregano or dried tarragon
- 1 medium-sized red onion, thinly sliced
- 4 garlic cloves, crushed
- 2 ½ cups of organic homemade low-sodium chicken stock
- 1 teaspoon of sea salt (to taste)
- 1 teaspoon of freshly ground black pepper (to taste)

Instructions:

- Season the pork steaks with salt and black pepper.
- Press the "Sauté" function on your Instant Pot.
- Once hot, add the pork steaks and cook for 5 minutes per side or until brown. Remove and set aside.
- Add the onions to your Instant Pot and sauté for 3 minutes or until softened, stirring occasionally. Add the garlic and sauté for another minute, stirring occasionally.
- Deglaze your Instant Pot with the chicken broth and scrape any brown bits on the bottom.
- Stir in the ½ pounds of Cremini mushrooms, Dijon mustard, 2 tablespoons of fresh lime juice, 1 tablespoon of dried oregano and place the pork on top.
- Add the sweet potatoes on top of the pork.
- Lock the lid and ensure the valve is closed. Press the "Manual" button and cook for 7 minutes on High Pressure. When the cooking is done, quick release any remaining pressure and carefully remove the lid.
- Remove the sweet potatoes and pork steaks.
- Press the "Sauté" function on your Instant Pot and stir in the unsweetened coconut cream with coconut flour. Allow the gravy to thicken, stirring occasionally.
- Ladle the sauce and mushrooms over the pork steaks and sweet potatoes.
- Serve and enjoy!

Nutrition information per serving:

- Calories: 424
- Fat: 9.3g
- Carbohydrates: 30.9g
- Dietary Fiber: 4.8g
- Protein: 52.5g

Happy Hawaiian-Inspired Pork

Time: 26 minutes
Servings: 8
Ingredients:

- 2 pounds of boneless organic pork shoulder cut into 1-inch pieces
- 2 tablespoons of olive oil
- 3 garlic cloves, finely minced
- 1 large red bell pepper, chopped
- 1 large yellow onion, finely chopped
- 3 cups of fresh pineapple chunks
- ½ cup of fresh pineapple juice
- 1 tablespoon of almond flour
- 2 tablespoons of low-sodium coconut aminos
- 1 1-inch fresh ginger, peeled and finely grated
- 1 teaspoon of sea salt (to taste)
- ½ teaspoon of freshly ground black pepper (to taste)
- 2 teaspoons of dried oregano
- ¼ cup of fresh cilantro, finely chopped

Instructions:

- In a bowl, add the pineapple juice, almond flour, coconut aminos, ginger, and garlic. Stir until well incorporated together.
- Press the "Sauté" function on your Instant Pot and add 1 tablespoon of olive oil.
- Once hot and ready, add the onions and red bell pepper. Sauté for 3 minutes or until softened, stirring occasionally. Remove and set aside.
- Add the remaining tablespoon of olive oil to your Instant Pot. Add the pork pieces to your Instant Pot and sauté until brown, stirring occasionally.
- Stir in the fresh pineapple chunks, dried oregano, salt, and black pepper.
- Stir in the pineapple juice mixture and give a good stir.
- Lock the lid and ensure the valve is closed. Press the "Manual" button and cook for 10 minutes on High Pressure.
- When the cooking is done, naturally release the pressure for 5 minutes and then quick release the remaining pressure. Carefully remove the lid.
- Stir in the softened onions and red bell peppers to your Instant Pot. Stir until well combined. Adjust the seasoning if necessary.
- Garnish with fresh cilantro.
- Serve and enjoy!

Nutrition information per serving:

- Calories: 398
- Fat: 28.3g
- Carbohydrates: 14.3g
- Dietary Fiber: 3g
- Protein: 23g

Highly Seasoned Barbacoa Beef Pot Roast

Time: 1 hour and 40 minutes

Servings: 8

Ingredients:

- 2 pounds of organic boneless beef chuck roast
- 2 tablespoons of olive oil, avocado oil, or coconut oil
- 1 medium-sized red onion, thinly sliced
- 1 medium-sized yellow bell pepper, sliced
- 1 medium-sized red bell pepper, sliced
- 1 jalapeno pepper, sliced
- 4 garlic cloves, crushed
- ½ cup of homemade low-sodium organic beef broth
- 1 (14.5-ounce) can of diced tomatoes, undrained
- 1 (7-ounce) can of chipotle peppers
- 1 tablespoon of sea salt
- 1 teaspoon of dried or fresh oregano
- 1 teaspoon of freshly ground black pepper
- 1 tablespoon of organic ground cumin
- 1 tablespoon of smoked paprika
- 1 teaspoon of organic cayenne pepper

Instructions:

- In a bowl, add and mix all the spices together until well incorporated.
- Rub the spice mixture over the beef chuck roast.
- Press the "Sauté" function on your Instant Pot and add 1 tablespoon of olive oil.
- Once hot and ready, add the beef chuck roast and cook for 3 minutes per side or until brown. Remove and set aside.
- Add the remaining tablespoon of olive oil to your Instant Pot. Add the onions, garlic, red bell pepper, yellow bell pepper, and jalapeno pepper. Sauté until softened, stirring occasionally.
- Add the beef broth, diced tomatoes, and chipotle peppers.
- Place the beef chuck roast on top of the vegetables.
- Lock the lid and ensure the valve is closed. Press the "Manual" button and cook for 45 minutes on High Pressure.
- When the cooking is done, quick release or naturally release the pressure. Carefully remove the lid.
- Transfer the beef chuck roast and shred using two forks. Return to your Instant Pot and stir until well combined.
- Serve and enjoy!

Nutrition information per serving:

- Calories: 273
- Fat: 10.9g
- Carbohydrates: 6.9g
- Dietary Fiber: 1.5g
- Protein: 36g

Lovely Cuban-Inspired Garlicky Pork

Time: 1 hour and 30 minutes

Servings: 6

Ingredients:

- 3 pounds of fresh boneless pork shoulder, well-trimmed and cut into large pieces
- 2 tablespoons of olive oil
- 6 garlic cloves
- 2/3 cup of fresh grapefruit juice
- 1/3 cup of fresh lime juice
- 1 tablespoon of fresh oregano, finely chopped
- 1 tablespoon of fresh parsley, finely chopped
- ½ tablespoon of organic ground cumin powder
- 1 tablespoon of paprika
- 1 bay leaf
- 1 tablespoon of grounded sea salt
- 1 teaspoon of freshly ground black pepper (to taste)

Instructions:

- In a blender, add the garlic, grapefruit juice, lime juice, olive oil, oregano, parsley, ground cumin powder, paprika, salt and black pepper. Blend until smooth.
- In a bowl, add the pork pieces and pour the marinade over the meat. Allow to marinate overnight.
- Add the pork pieces and the marinade to your Instant Pot. Add the bay leaf.
- Lock the lid and ensure the valve is closed. Press the "Manual" button and cook for 70 minutes on High Pressure.
- When the cooking is done, allow for a full natural release method. Carefully remove the lid.
- Transfer the pork pieces to a serving platter and shred using two forks.
- Return the pork pieces to your Instant Pot. Press "Sauté" function on your Instant Pot and allow to simmer until the liquid is reduced by half.
- Serve and enjoy!

Nutrition information per serving:

- Calories: 215
- Fat: 9.6g
- Carbohydrates: 2.7g
- Dietary Fiber: 0.3g
- Protein: 25.3g

Enjoyable Teriyaki Pork Tenderloin

Time: 20 minutes

Servings: 4

Ingredients:

* 2 pounds of pork tenderloins
* 2 tablespoon of olive oil
* ½ cup of low-sodium coconut aminos
* 1 cup of fresh pineapple juice
* 1/3 cup of fresh lime juice
* 1 tablespoon of sesame oil
* 1 teaspoon of apple cider vinegar
* A small pinch of crushed red pepper flakes
* 1 teaspoon of organic ground ginger powder
* 1 tablespoon of almond flour
* 1 teaspoon of garlic powder
* 1 teaspoon of onion powder
* 1 teaspoon of sea salt (to taste)
* 1 teaspoon of freshly ground black pepper (to taste)

Instructions:

* Press the "Sauté" function on your Instant Pot and add the olive oil.
* Once hot, working in batches if necessary, add the pork tenderloins and sear for 2 minutes on each side until brown. Turn off the "Sauté" setting.
* Add the coconut aminos, apple cider vinegar, lime juice, pineapple juice, sesame oil, crushed red pepper flakes, ground ginger powder, garlic powder, onion powder, salt, and black pepper.
* Lock the lid and ensure the valve is closed. Press the "Manual" button and cook for 9 minutes on High Pressure.
* When the cooking is done, naturally release the pressure for 10 minutes, and then quick release the remaining pressure. Carefully remove the lid.
* Remove the pork tenderloins.
* Press the "Sauté" function on your Instant Pot and sprinkle with almond flour. Allow to simmer until thickened, stirring occasionally.
* Spoon the sauce over the tenderloins.
* Serve and enjoy!

Nutrition information per serving:

* Calories: 428
* Fat: 16g
* Carbohydrates: 10.4g
* Dietary Fiber: 0.2g
* Protein: 59.7g

Invincible Beef Roast with Whole30 BBQ and Coleslaw

Time: 50 minutes
Servings: 6
Ingredients:

- 3 pounds of fresh boneless beef chuck roast, cut into 4 large separate pieces
- 2 tablespoons of olive oil
- 1 large yellow or red onion, thinly sliced
- ½ cup of organic tomato paste
- 2 tablespoons of organic homemade Dijon mustard (if using store-bought make sure to check ingredients)
- 4 garlic cloves, minced
- 1 tablespoon of dried oregano
- 1 cup of homemade low-sodium organic beef stock or plain water
- 1 tablespoon of chili powder
- 1 tablespoon of regular or smoked paprika
- 1 tablespoon of almond flour
- 1 tablespoon of sea salt (to taste)
- 1 teaspoon of freshly ground black pepper (to taste)
- 1 tablespoon of apple cider vinegar

Coleslaw Mix Ingredients:

- ¼ medium-sized green cabbage, cored and shredded
- ¼ medium-sized red cabbage, cored and shredded
- 2 large fresh orange carrots, peeled and finely grated
- ¼ cup of fresh parsley leaves, finely chopped
- ½ cup of fresh pineapple chunks
- ¼ cup of white wine vinegar
- ½ cup of homemade Whole30-friendly mayonnaise
- ½ teaspoon of sea salt

Instructions:

- Press the "Sauté" function on your Instant Pot and add the olive oil.
- Once hot, add the thinly sliced red onions and garlic cloves. Sauté for 2 minutes, stirring occasionally.
- Add the chuck roast and cook for 4 to 6 minutes until brown on all sides. Turn off "Sauté" function on your Instant Pot.
- In a bowl, mix the remaining beef roast ingredients
- In a large bowl, add the tomato paste, Dijon mustard, oregano, beef stock, chili powder, paprika, almond flour, salt, black pepper, and apple cider vinegar. Mix well.
- Pour over the beef chuck roast and onions. You can give a good stir if needed.

- Lock the lid and ensure the valve is closed. Press the "Manual" button and cook for 44 minutes on High Pressure.
- Meanwhile, in a large bowl, add all the coleslaw ingredients and stir until well incorporated.
- When the cooking is done, naturally release the pressure for 10 minutes and then quick release the remaining pressure. Carefully remove the lid.
- Transfer the chuck roast to a serving platter and shred using two forks.
- Sprinkle the almond flour to the liquid in your Instant Pot. Allow the liquid to thicken.
- Stir the shredded beef to your Instant Pot until well coated with the liquid.
- Serve and enjoy with coleslaw.

Nutrition information per serving:

- Calories: 500
- Fat: 19.5g
- Carbohydrates: 7.1g
- Dietary Fiber: 2.7g
- Protein: 70.8g

Exciting Beef Ragu

Time: 1 hour   Servings: 4

Ingredients:

- 1 ½ pounds of chuck roast or chuck steak, cut into large separated pieces
- 1 teaspoon of sea salt (to taste)
- 1 teaspoon of freshly ground white pepper (to taste)
- 1 medium-sized fresh celery stalk, finely chopped
- 1 large orange carrot, cut into 1-inch pieces
- 1 medium-sized yellow onion, finely chopped
- 4 garlic cloves, minced
- 2 bay leaves
- 1 teaspoon of regular or smoked paprika
- 1 teaspoon of dried oregano
- 1 teaspoon of dried thyme
- 1 teaspoon of dried basil
- ½ teaspoon of ground organic cinnamon powder
- 1 fresh red chili, minced
- 1 (15-ounce) can of diced tomatoes
- 1 tablespoon of low-sodium coconut aminos
- 1 cup of homemade low-sodium beef broth

Instructions:

- Press the "Sauté" function on your Instant Pot and add the olive oil.
- Once hot and ready, add the finely chopped yellow onions, carrot pieces, finely chopped celery, red chili, salt, and pepper. Sauté for 4 to 6 minutes or until softened, stirring occasionally.
- Add the steak to your Instant Pot along with the remaining ingredients. Give a good stir.
- Lock the lid and ensure the valve is closed. Press the "Manual" button and cook for 30 minutes on High Pressure.
- When the timer beeps, naturally release the pressure for 10 minutes and then quick release the remaining pressure. Carefully remove the lid.
- Press the "Sauté" function on your Instant Pot and use a potato masher to mash beef the pieces into tiny pieces. Allow to cook in your Instant Pot for around 10 minutes or until the liquid thickens, stirring occasionally.
- Serve and enjoy!

Nutrition information per serving:

- Calories: 408
- Fat: 14.7g
- Carbohydrates: 7g
- Dietary Fiber: 1.8g
- Protein: 58.7g

Unstoppable Pulled Pork with Whole30 Friendly Barbecue Sauce

Time: 2 hours   Servings: 10

Ingredients:

- 1 (5 pounds) organic fresh boneless or bone-in pork shoulder, cut into 2 pieces
- 2 tablespoons of olive oil, coconut oil, or avocado oil
- 2 cups of homemade low-sodium chicken stock
- 1 tablespoon of garlic powder or 4 minced garlic cloves
- 1 tablespoon of onion powder
- 1 tablespoon of chili powder
- 1 tablespoon of smoked paprika powder
- 1 teaspoon of organic ground cayenne pepper
- 1 tablespoon of sea salt (more to taste)
- 1 tablespoon of freshly ground black pepper (more to taste)

Whole30-Friendly Barbecue Sauce Ingredients:

- ½ cup of fresh organic tomato paste
- 6 dates, soaked in lukewarm water for 15 minutes
- 2 garlic cloves, minced
- 1 tablespoon of chili powder
- ½ cup of low-sodium coconut aminos

Instructions:

- In a bowl, add the garlic powder, onion powder, chili powder, smoked paprika powder, ground cayenne pepper, salt, and black pepper. Mix well.
- Rub the seasoning mix over the pork pieces.
- Press the "Sauté" function on your Instant Pot and add the olive oil.
- Once the display reads hot, add the pork pieces and sear until brown on both sides.
- Add the chicken stock to your Instant Pot.
- Lock the lid and ensure the valve is closed. Select the "Manual" button and cook for 90 minutes on High Pressure.
- When the timer beeps, naturally release the pressure and carefully remove the lid.
- Transfer the pork pieces to a serving platter and shred using two forks. Return the shredded pork to the liquid and stir until well combined. Adjust the seasoning as needed.
- In a blender, add all the Whole30-friendly barbecue sauce ingredients and blend until smooth. Drizzle the barbecue sauce over the shredded pork. Serve and enjoy!

Nutrition information per serving:

- Calories: 380
- Fat: 11g
- Carbohydrates: 7.4g
- Dietary Fiber: 1g
- Protein: 60.2g

Millionaire Beef and Broccoli

Time: 29 minutes
Servings: 6
Ingredients:

- 2 pounds of flank steak, thinly sliced
- 2 tablespoons of olive oil
- 2 tablespoons of sesame oil
- 4 garlic cloves, minced
- 1 tablespoon of almond flour
- 4 cups of fresh broccoli florets
- 1 cup of homemade low-sodium organic beef stock
- ½ cup of low-sodium coconut aminos
- 1 teaspoon of onion powder
- 1 teaspoon of sea salt (to taste)
- ½ teaspoon of crushed red pepper flakes
- 1 cup of ordinary warm water
- Toasted sesame seeds (to serve)
- Freshly sliced green onions (to serve)

Instructions:

- Press the "Sauté" function on your Instant Pot and add the olive oil.
- In a microwavable safe bowl, add the broccoli and fill 1 cup of water. Microwave for 2 minutes and 30 seconds until almost steamed. Discard the water and set aside.
- Once the display reads hot on your Instant Pot, working in batches, add the beef slices and sear for 1 minute per side. Remove and set aside.
- Add the garlic to your Instant Pot and sauté for 1 minute or until fragrant, stirring occasionally.
- Stir in the 1 cup of beef stock, ½ cup of low-sodium coconut aminos, 2 tablespoons of sesame oil, and seasonings. Stir until well combined.
- Gently stir in the beef slices.
- Lock the lid and ensure the valve is closed. Press the "Manual" button and cook for 10 minutes on High Pressure.
- When the cooking is done, quick release the pressure and carefully remove the lid.
- Sprinkle the 1 tablespoon of almond flour and stir in the broccoli. Allow to cook until thickened, stirring occasionally.
- Transfer the beef and broccoli to a serving platter. Allow the liquid in your Instant Pot to simmer until it thickens even more.
- Spoon the sauce over the beef and broccoli.
- Top with toasted sesame seeds and sliced green onions.
- Serve and enjoy!

Nutrition information per serving:

- Calories: 409
- Fat: 22.3g
- Carbohydrates: 6.4g
- Dietary Fiber: 1.8g
- Protein: 44g

Superstar Mushroom and Steak Stroganoff

Time: 20 minutes   Servings: 6

Ingredients:

- 2 pounds of beef steak, well-trimmed and thinly sliced into strips
- 2 cups of cremini mushrooms, brown mushrooms, or Swiss button mushrooms, sliced
- 4 garlic cloves, minced
- 1 large onion, finely chopped
- 2 tablespoons of olive oil, coconut oil, or avocado oil
- ¼ cup of organic fresh tomato paste
- 1 tablespoon of organic homemade Dijon mustard (if using store-bought make sure you check ingredients)
- 1 fresh bay leaf
- 1 cup of homemade low-sodium beef stock
- 1 tablespoon of almond flour
- ½ cup of unsweetened coconut cream
- 2 tablespoons of fresh parsley leaves, finely chopped
- 1 tablespoon of sea salt (to taste)
- 1 teaspoon of freshly ground black pepper (to taste)

Instructions:

- Press the "Sauté" function on your Instant Pot and add the oil.
- Once hot, add the finely chopped onions. Sauté for 2 minutes or until lightly browned, stirring occasionally.
- Add the beef strips and cook for 3 to 4 minutes or until browned.
- Stir in the 2 cups of mushrooms, minced garlic cloves, ¼ cup of tomato paste, organic Dijon mustard, 1 bay leaf, and 1 cup of beef stock. Give a good stir.
- Lock the lid and ensure the valve is closed. Press the "Manual" button and cook for 10 minutes on High Pressure.
- When the cooking is done, allow to sit for 5 minutes, and then quick release the remaining pressure. Carefully remove the lid.
- Discard the bay leaf.
- Press "Sauté" function on your Instant Pot and sprinkle the almond flour. Allow to simmer until slightly thickened.
- Stir in the unsweetened coconut cream, fresh parsley, salt, and black pepper. Turn off "Sauté" function and allow to cool.
- Serve and enjoy!

Nutrition information per serving:

- Calories: 399
- Fat: 17.5g
- Carbohydrates: 2.4g
- Dietary Fiber: 0.9g

- Protein: 56.1g

Worldwide Famous Whole30 Chili

Time: 1 hour
Servings: 8
Ingredients:

- 1 pound of extra-lean grass-fed ground beef
- 2 tablespoons of olive oil, coconut oil, or avocado oil
- 1 medium-sized red onion, finely chopped
- 1 large sweet potato, cut into bite-sized pieces
- 1 medium-sized fresh bell pepper, finely chopped
- 1 medium-sized fresh red bell pepper, finely chopped
- 1 medium-sized fresh Jalapeno pepper, finely chopped
- 2 cups of finely chopped cauliflower florets
- 1 ½ cups of organic homemade pumpkin puree OR 1 (15-ounce) can of pure pumpkin puree
- 1 (14.5-ounce) can of diced tomatoes, undrained
- 2 cups of homemade low-sodium organic chicken stock OR beef broth
- Chopped avocado (for topping)
- Freshly chopped cilantro (for topping)
- Non-plain yogurt (for topping)

Chili Seasoning Ingredients:

- 1 tablespoon of sea salt (to taste)
- 1 teaspoon of freshly ground black pepper (to taste)
- 3 heaping tablespoons of organic chili powder (any brand)
- 2 tablespoons of regular paprika or smoked paprika
- 1 tablespoon of organic ground cumin powder
- 1 tablespoon of dried basil
- 1 tablespoon of dried parsley
- 1 teaspoon of organic ground cinnamon powder
- 1 teaspoon of onion powder
- 1 teaspoon of garlic powder
- 1 teaspoon of organic cayenne pepper

Instructions:

- In a small bowl, add all the chili seasoning ingredients and mix well.
- Press the "Sauté" function on your Instant Pot and add the cooking oil.
- Once the oil is hot and ready, add the beef and red onions. Cook until the ground beef has browned and the onions have softened, this will take around 7 minutes.
- Add the bell peppers, jalapeno pepper, cauliflower, pumpkin puree, diced tomatoes, sweet potato, and chicken stock.
- Add the chili seasoning mix and give a good stir.

- Lock the lid and ensure the valve is sealed. Press the "Manual" button and cook for 9 minutes.
- When the cooking is done, naturally release the pressure and carefully remove the lid.
- Adjust the seasoning if necessary
- Spoon the chili to serving bowls and add the desired toppings.
- Serve and enjoy!

Nutrition information per serving:

- Calories: 278
- Fat: 12g
- Carbohydrates: 19.35g
- Dietary Fiber: 7.8g
- Protein: 23.4g

Extremely Popular Red Wine Pot Roast with Winter Vegetables

Time: 1 hour and 30 minutes   Servings: 6

Ingredients:

- 3 pounds of grass-fed chuck roast
- 3 tablespoons of olive oil, avocado oil, or coconut oil
- 1 pound of large fresh orange carrots, peeled and cut into bite-sized pieces
- 2 medium-sized parsnips, peeled and cut into 1-inch pieces
- 4 medium-sized celery stalks, chopped
- 1 cup of Portobello mushrooms, sliced
- 2 large yellow or white onions, thinly sliced
- 6 garlic cloves, minced
- ¼ cup of organic tomato paste
- 1 cup of red wine
- 3 cups of homemade low-sodium beef stock
- 2 fresh sprigs of thyme
- 1 fresh sprig of rosemary
- 3 tablespoons of almond flour
- 1 tablespoon of fresh parsley, finely chopped
- 3 bay leaves
- 1 teaspoon of onion powder
- 1 teaspoon of garlic powder
- 1 tablespoon of sea salt (more to taste)
- 1 tablespoon of freshly ground black pepper (to taste)

Instructions:

- Season the chuck roast with salt, black pepper, onion powder, and garlic powder.
- Press the "Sauté" function on your Instant Pot and add 2 tablespoons of olive oil.
- Once hot, add the chuck roast and sear on both sides for 3 minutes until brown. Remove and set aside.
- Add the remaining tablespoon of olive oil and all the vegetables (carrots, parsnips, celery, mushrooms, onion, and garlic) to your Instant Pot and sauté for around 3 minutes, stirring occasionally. Stir in the tomato paste, red wine, and beef stock.
- Return the chuck roast to your Instant Pot.
- Place the fresh sprigs of thyme, a fresh sprig of rosemary, finely chopped parsley, and bay leaves to your Instant Pot.
- Lock the lid and ensure the valve is closed. Select the "Manual" button and cook for 60 minutes on High Pressure.
- When the cooking is done, naturally release the pressure and carefully remove the lid.
- Remove the chuck roast from your Instant Pot and discard the bay leaves.
- Press the "Sauté" function on your Instant Pot and sprinkle the almond flour. Allow to simmer until the vegetables and the liquid thickened.
- Serve the pot roast with the winter vegetables. Serve and enjoy!

Nutrition information per serving:

- Calories: 532
- Fat: 29.3g
- Carbohydrates: 15g
- Dietary Fiber: 2.9g
- Protein: 48g

Chapter 7: Vegan and Vegetarian Recipes

Hearty Spaghetti Squash Cauliflower Alfredo

Time: 28 minutes   Servings: 6

Ingredients:

- 1 large fresh whole spaghetti squash, cut in half
- 1 cup of water
- 2 cups of fresh cauliflower, chopped
- 2 cups of fresh broccoli, chopped
- 1 tablespoon of coconut or almond flour
- 2 tablespoon of ghee

Vegan Cauliflower Sauce Ingredients:

- 2 cups of cashews, soaked
- 1 ½ to 2 cups of unsweetened coconut milk or almond milk
- Juice from a ½ fresh lemon
- 8 garlic cloves
- 1 tablespoon of ghee
- A pinch of cayenne pepper
- 1 teaspoon of sea salt
- 1 teaspoon of freshly ground black pepper

Instructions:

- Add all the vegan cauliflower sauce ingredients to a food processor and pulse until smooth and creamy.
- Add 1 cup of water and a trivet or steamer rack to your Instant Pot.
- Place the spaghetti squash halves on top of the trivet.
- Close and seal the lid on your Instant Pot. Select the "Manual" button and cook for 6 minutes on High Pressure.
- When the cooking is done, naturally release the pressure for 5 minutes and then quick release the remaining pressure. Carefully remove the lid and the spaghetti squash halves.
- Shred the spaghetti squash halves using two forks and discard the water from your Instant Pot. Remove the trivet.
- Press the "Sauté" function on your Instant Pot and add the ghee.
- Once the ghee has melted, add the cauliflower and broccoli. Sauté for 3 minutes or until softened, stirring occasionally.
- Stir in the vegan cauliflower sauce to your Instant Pot and cook until well heated through. Sprinkle flour over the alfredo sauce and cook until thick.
- Spoon the cauliflower-broccoli alfredo sauce over the spaghetti squash. Enjoy!

Nutrition information per serving:

- Calories: 811
- Fat: 70.8g
- Carbohydrates: 40.3g
- Dietary Fiber: 7.5g
- Protein: 16.4g

You Will Love These Vegan Stuffed Bell Peppers

Time: 20 minutes   Servings: 4

Ingredients:

- 4 large sweet bell peppers, any color, tops removed, and inner portions scooped out
- 2 tablespoons of coconut oil, melted
- 1 cup of cauliflower rice
- 4 garlic cloves, minced
- 1 medium-sized fresh zucchini, finely chopped
- 1 (14.5-ounce) can of diced tomatoes, undrained
- 1 medium-sized sweet potato, peeled and cut into cubes
- 1 medium fresh jalapeno pepper, finely chopped
- 1 teaspoon of dried basil
- 1 cup of fresh kale, roughly chopped
- ½ teaspoon of crushed red pepper flakes
- 2 teaspoons of smoked paprika
- 1 teaspoon of organic ground cumin powder
- 1 tablespoon of fresh lime juice
- 1 teaspoon of sea salt (to taste)
- 1 teaspoon of freshly ground black pepper (to taste)
- 1 ripe avocado, chopped (for garnishing)
- Fresh chopped cilantro (for garnishing)

Instructions:

- Brush 1 tablespoon of melted coconut oil over the sweet bell peppers.
- Press the "Sauté" function on your Instant Pot and add the remaining tablespoon of coconut oil.
- Once hot and ready, add the onions, garlic, zucchini, and jalapeno pepper. Sauté for 4 minutes or until almost softened, stirring occasionally.
- Add the sweet potatoes and sauté for 2 minutes more, stirring occasionally.
- Turn off "Sauté" function and transfer the contents to a large bowl.
- Add the diced tomatoes, basil, kale, cauliflower rice, oregano, crushed red pepper flakes, smoked paprika, cumin powder, lime juice, salt, and black pepper. Stir until well combined.
- Fill the bell peppers with the vegetable mixture.
- Add 1 cup of water and a trivet to your Instant Pot.
- Place the bell peppers on top of the Instant Pot.
- Close and seal the lid on your Instant Pot. Press the "Manual" button and cook for 6 minutes on High Pressure.
- When the cooking is done, quick release the pressure and carefully remove the lid.
- Remove the bell peppers from your Instant Pot and allow to cool.
- Top with fresh cilantro and chopped avocado. Serve and enjoy!

Nutrition information per serving:

- Calories: 164
- Fat: 7.3g
- Carbohydrates: 23.8g
- Dietary Fiber: 5.3g
- Protein: 4.3g

Flavorful Cauliflower Tikka Masala

Time: 28 minutes
Servings: 7
Ingredients:

- 1 large cauliflower head, chopped into florets
- ½ cup of unsweetened coconut cream
- 2 tablespoons of ghee
- 1 1-inch fresh ginger, finely grated
- 1 medium-sized red onion, finely chopped
- 4 garlic cloves, minced
- 1 teaspoon of organic ground turmeric powder
- 1 teaspoon of chili powder
- 1 teaspoons of organic dried fenugreek leaves
- 1 teaspoon of ground cumin
- 1 tablespoon of organic garam masala
- 1 (28-ounce) can of diced tomatoes, undrained
- 1 teaspoon of sea salt (to taste)
- 1 teaspoon of freshly ground black pepper (to taste)

Instructions:

- Press the "Sauté" function on your Instant Pot and add the ghee.
- Once hot, add the ginger, garlic, and red onions to your Instant Pot. Sauté for 5 minutes or until softened, stirring occasionally.
- Stir in all the spices and sauté for 1 minute to release the aroma, stirring occasionally. Turn off "Sauté" function.
- Stir in the diced tomatoes and cauliflower to your Instant Pot.
- Close and seal the lid on your Instant Pot. Press the "Manual" button and cook for 2 minutes on High Pressure.
- When the cooking is done, quick release the pressure and remove the lid.
- Stir in the coconut cream and adjust the seasoning as needed.
- Serve and enjoy!

Nutrition information per serving:

- Calories: 135
- Fat: 8.2g
- Carbohydrates: 11.7g
- Dietary Fiber: 4.8g
- Protein: 3.8g

Welcoming Sautéed Lemon-Garlic Kale

Time: 10 minutes
Servings: 4
Ingredients:

- 1 large bunch of kale, roughly chopped (around 6 cups)
- 3 tablespoons of ghee
- 1 fresh medium-sized lemon, juice
- 4 garlic cloves, minced
- 1/8 teaspoon of cayenne pepper
- 1 teaspoon of sea salt (to taste)
- ½ teaspoon of freshly ground black pepper (to taste)

Instructions:

- Press the "Sauté" function on your Instant Pot and add the ghee.
- Once hot, add the kale, lemon juice, and garlic.
- Sauté for 5 minutes or until slightly wilted, stirring occasionally.
- Sprinkle with salt, black pepper, and a pinch of cayenne pepper.
- Serve and enjoy!

Nutrition information per serving:

- Calories: 143
- Fat: 9.6g
- Carbohydrates: 12.8g
- Dietary Fiber: 2g
- Protein: 3.4g

Glorious Brussel Sprouts with Pecans

Time: 15 minutes
Servings: 4
Ingredients:

- 1 pound of fresh baby Brussel sprouts
- ¼ cup of homemade low-sodium vegetable stock
- ½ teaspoon of onion powder
- 1 teaspoon of sea salt (to taste)
- ½ teaspoon of freshly ground black pepper (to taste)
- ½ cup of pecans, roughly chopped
- ½ teaspoon of ground cinnamon powder

Instructions:

- Add the Brussel sprouts and vegetable stock to your Instant Pot.
- Close and seal the lid on your Instant Pot. Press the "Manual" button and cook for 2 minutes on High Pressure.
- When the cooking is done, quick release the pressure and carefully remove the lid.
- Press the "Sauté" function on your Instant Pot and add the pecans. Sprinkle onion powder, salt, black pepper, and cinnamon.
- Allow to simmer or until the liquid is reduced by half.
- Serve and enjoy!

Nutrition information per serving:

- Calories: 195
- Fat: 15.4g
- Carbohydrates: 13.3g
- Dietary Fiber: 6.5g
- Protein: 6.1g

Appetizing Herb-Buttered Carrots

Time: 15 minutes

Servings: 6

Ingredients:

- 2 pounds of fresh orange baby carrots
- 1 cup of homemade low-sodium vegetable stock
- 4 tablespoons of ghee or coconut butter
- 2 sprigs of fresh thyme
- 2 sprigs of fresh dill
- 1 tablespoon of fresh oregano, finely chopped
- 1 tablespoon of fresh parsley, finely chopped
- 1 teaspoon of sea salt (to taste)
- 1 teaspoon of freshly ground black pepper (to taste)

Instructions:

- Add all the ingredients to your Instant Pot except for the ghee and herbs.
- Close and seal the lid on your Instant Pot. Press the "Manual" button and cook for 4 minutes on High Pressure.
- When the cooking is done, quick release the pressure and carefully remove the lid.
- Press the "Sauté" function on your Instant Pot and add the ghee and herbs.
- Sauté for around 2 minutes, stirring occasionally.
- Serve and enjoy!

Nutrition information per serving:

- Calories: 137
- Fat: 8.5g
- Carbohydrates: 14.9g
- Dietary Fiber: 3.7g
- Protein: 1.7g

Healthy and Delicious Borscht

Time: 1 hour and 25 minutes
Servings: 8
Ingredients:

- ½ pounds of orange carrots, finely grated
- 1 medium-sized red onion, finely chopped
- 3 medium-sized beets, peeled and chopped into bite-sized pieces
- 6 medium-sized potatoes, cut into bite-sized pieces
- ½ large cabbage head, cored and finely shredded
- 2 tablespoons of tomato paste
- 6 cups of homemade low-sodium vegetable stock
- 3 garlic cloves, minced
- 1 tablespoon of olive oil
- 1 teaspoon of sea salt (to taste)
- 1 teaspoon of freshly ground black pepper (to taste)

Instructions:

- Press the "Sauté" function on your Instant Pot and add the olive oil.
- Once hot, add the onions, garlic, and grated carrots. Sauté for 4 to 6 minutes or until softened, stirring occasionally.
- Add all the remaining ingredients to your Instant Pot.
- Close and seal the lid on your Instant Pot. Press the "Manual" button and cook for 14 minutes on High Pressure.
- When the cooking is done, quick release the pressure and carefully remove the lid.
- Give the borscht a good stir and adjust the seasoning as needed.
- Serve and enjoy!

Nutrition information per serving:

- Calories: 163
- Fat: 3.4g
- Carbohydrates: 29g
- Dietary Fiber: 5.7g
- Protein: 6.4g

Yawning Mashed Cauliflower

Time: 8 minutes

Servings: 6

Ingredients:

- 2 large cauliflower heads, cored and roughly chopped into florets
- 2 ½ cups of homemade low-sodium vegetable stock
- ½ cup of unsweetened coconut cream
- ¼ cup of ghee or coconut butter
- 4 garlic cloves, minced
- 2 tablespoons of sesame seeds
- 2 tablespoons fresh parsley, finely chopped
- 1 teaspoon of sea salt (to taste)
- 1 teaspoon of freshly ground black pepper (to taste)

Instructions:

- Add the vegetable stock and cauliflower florets to your Instant Pot.
- Close and seal the lid. Press the "Manual" button and cook for 3 minutes on High Pressure.
- When the cooking is done, quick release the pressure and carefully remove the lid.
- Press the "Sauté" function on your Instant Pot and set to the lowest temperature.
- Stir in the ghee, coconut cream, garlic, sea salt, black pepper, 1 tablespoon of sesame seeds, and 1 tablespoon of parsley.
- Use an immersion blender to blend the cauliflower until smooth.
- Top with remaining sesame seeds and parsley.
- Serve and enjoy!

Nutrition information per serving:

- Calories: 185
- Fat: 12g
- Carbohydrates: 7.3g
- Dietary Fiber: 1.3g
- Protein: 12.3g

Exotic Vegan Chili

Time: 23 minutes
Servings: 8
Ingredients:

- 2 tablespoons of olive oil, coconut oil, coconut oil, or ghee
- 1 medium-sized red onion, finely chopped
- 4 garlic cloves, minced
- 3 medium celery stalks, finely chopped
- 2 medium carrots, finely chopped
- 1 (28-ounce) can) of crushed tomatoes, undrained
- 2 cups of low-sodium organic vegetable stock
- 1 medium-sized sweet green bell pepper, finely chopped
- 1 medium-sized sweet red bell pepper, finely chopped
- 1 medium-sized sweet potato, cut into bite-sized pieces
- 1 pound of butternut squash, cut into bite-sized pieces
- 1 tablespoon of chili powder
- 1 teaspoon of organic ground cumin powder
- ½ teaspoon of organic ground cinnamon powder
- 1 teaspoon of cayenne pepper powder
- 1 teaspoon of salt (to taste)
- 1 teaspoon of freshly ground black pepper (to taste)
- ½ cup of fresh cilantro, finely chopped (For serving)
- Avocado slices (For serving)

Instructions:

- Press the "Sauté" function on your Instant Pot and add the oil.
- Once the display reads hot, add the onion, garlic, celery, carrots, bell peppers, and butternut squash. Sauté for 4 to 6 minutes or until softened, stirring occasionally.
- Add the remaining ingredients to your Instant Pot except for the fresh cilantro and avocado slices.
- Lock the lid and ensure the valve is closed. Press the "Manual" button and cook for 12 minutes on High Pressure.
- When the cooking is done, allow to release the pressure naturally for 5 minutes, and then quick release the remaining pressure. Carefully remove the lid.
- Ladle the chili into serving bowls and top with cilantro and avocado slices.
- Serve and enjoy!

Nutrition information per serving:

- Calories: 263
- Fat: 11.5g
- Carbohydrates: 16g
- Dietary Fiber: 4g
- Protein: 17g

Honorable Yukon Potato Curry

Time: 50 minutes
Servings: 6
Ingredients:

- 6 cups of Yukon potatoes, cut into bite-sized pieces
- 2 cups of fresh green beans, cut into bite-sized pieces
- 2 tablespoons of ghee
- 1 cup of unsweetened coconut cream
- 1 medium-sized red onion, finely chopped
- 4 garlic cloves, minced
- 2 tablespoons of organic curry powder
- 2 cups of low-sodium homemade vegetable stock
- 1 teaspoon of smoked paprika
- ½ teaspoon of organic cayenne pepper
- 3 tablespoons of almond flour
- 1 teaspoon of sea salt (to taste)
- 1 teaspoon of freshly ground black pepper (to taste)

Instructions:

- Press the "Sauté" function on your Instant Pot and add the ghee.
- Once hot, add the onions and garlic. Sauté until translucent, stirring occasionally.
- Turn off the "Sauté" function. Add the remaining ingredients to your Instant Pot except for the green beans, almond flour, and coconut cream.
- Close and seal the lid on your Instant Pot. Press the "Manual" button and cook for 20 minutes on High Pressure.
- When the cooking is done, naturally release the pressure and carefully remove the lid.
- Press the "Sauté" function on your Instant Pot and sprinkle with almond flour. Allow to simmer until thickened, stirring occasionally.
- Stir in the green beans and coconut cream to your Instant Pot. Allow to simmer for another 5 minutes or until tender, stirring occasionally
- Serve and enjoy!

Nutrition information per serving:

- Calories: 285
- Fat: 6g
- Carbohydrates: 48.6g
- Dietary Fiber: 9.2g
- Protein: 6.3g

Chapter 8: Savory Appetizers and Side Dishes Recipes

Enchanting Sautéed Garlic Artichokes

Time: 10 minutes
Servings: 4
Ingredients:

- 4 medium-sized artichokes hearts, trimmed and chopped
- 4 garlic cloves, minced
- 3 tablespoons of olive oil or coconut oil
- ½ fresh lemon, juice
- ¼ cup of fresh parsley leaves, finely chopped
- 1 teaspoon of sea salt (to taste)
- 1 teaspoon of freshly ground black pepper (to taste)

Instructions:

- Press the "Sauté" function on your Instant Pot and add the olive oil or coconut oil.
- Once the display reads hot, add the garlic and sauté until fragrant, stirring occasionally.
- Add the artichoke and sauté for 5 minutes or until golden, stirring occasionally.
- Season with salt and black pepper.
- Stir in the lemon juice and parsley.
- Turn off "Sauté" function on your Instant Pot and allow to cool.
- Serve and enjoy!

Nutrition information per serving:

- Calories: 171
- Fat: 10.8g
- Carbohydrates: 18g
- Dietary Fiber: 8.8g
- Protein: 5.5g

Out of This World Bratwurst and Cabbage

Time: 20 minutes

Servings: 8

Ingredients:

- 1 pound of bratwursts, cut into bite-sized pieces
- 2 large red onions, finely chopped
- 1 large green bell pepper, deseeded and chopped into chunks
- 1 medium-sized fresh green cabbage, shredded
- 1 medium-sized fresh red cabbage, shredded
- 4 garlic cloves, minced
- 1 cup of homemade low-sodium organic chicken broth
- 1 (14.5-ounce) can of crushed tomatoes, undrained
- 3 tablespoons of olive oil
- 1 teaspoon of sea salt (to taste)
- 1 teaspoon of freshly ground black pepper (to taste)

Instructions:

- Press the "Sauté" function on your Instant Pot and add the olive oil.
- Once hot, add the garlic and onions. Sauté until the onions are lightly browned, stirring occasionally.
- Add the bratwursts and sauté until lightly browned, stirring occasionally.
- Add the green cabbage, red cabbage, chicken broth, crushed tomatoes, salt, and black pepper to your Instant Pot.
- Close and seal the lid on your Instant Pot. Press the "Manual" button on your Instant Pot and cook for 6 minutes on High Pressure.
- When the cooking is done, naturally release the pressure and carefully remove the lid.
- Stir the bratwurst and cabbage combination until well combined.
- Serve and enjoy!

Nutrition information per serving:

- Calories: 318
- Fat: 22.2g
- Carbohydrates: 21g
- Dietary Fiber: 7.1g
- Protein: 11.8g

Desirable Brussel Sprouts with Mango and Nuts

Time: 18 minutes
Servings: 4
Ingredients:

- 1 pound of fresh Brussel sprouts, trimmed and chopped
- ½ cup of pecans, toasted and roughly chopped
- ½ cup of fresh mango cubes
- ¼ cup of fresh pineapple juice
- Juice from a ½ fresh lime
- 2 tablespoons of low-sodium coconut aminos
- 1 teaspoon of sea salt
- ½ teaspoon of freshly ground black pepper

Instructions:

- Add pineapple juice, lime juice, coconut aminos, and brussel sprouts to your Instant Pot. Sprinkle with salt and pepper.
- Close and seal the lid on your Instant Pot. Press the "Manual" button and cook for 3 minutes on High Pressure.
- When the cooking is done, quick release or naturally release the pressure. Remove the lid.
- Transfer the brussel sprouts to a large bowl.
- Add the roughly chopped pecans and fresh mango cubes. Stir until well combined.
- Serve and enjoy!

Nutrition information per serving:

- Calories: 172
- Fat: 10.6g
- Carbohydrates: 18.4g
- Dietary Fiber: 6.1g
- Protein: 5.7g

Exquisite Kale and Carrots with Bacon

Time: 27 minutes

Servings: 6

Ingredients:

- 4 cups of fresh kale, roughly chopped
- 6 bacon slices, cooked and chopped
- 4 medium-sized orange carrots, peeled and cut into slices
- 5 garlic cloves, minced
- 1 cup of homemade organic low-sodium chicken broth
- 1 tablespoon of balsamic vinegar
- 1 medium-sized red onion, thinly sliced
- 3 tablespoons of ghee
- A pinch of cayenne pepper
- 1 teaspoon of sea salt (to taste)
- 1 teaspoon of freshly ground black pepper (to taste)

Instructions:

- Press the "Sauté" function on your Instant Pot and add the ghee.
- Once the display reads hot, add the onion red onion and carrots to your Instant Pot. Saute for 3 to 4 minutes or until softened, stirring occasionally.
- Add the garlic and sauté for 30 seconds or until fragrant, stirring occasionally.
- Add the remaining ingredients to your Instant Pot and stir until well combined.
- Lock the lid and ensure the valve is closed. Press the "Manual" button and cook for 5 minutes on High Pressure.
- When the cooking is done, quick release the pressure and carefully remove the lid.
- Give the contents a good stir and adjust the seasoning as needed.
- Serve and enjoy!

Nutrition information per serving:

- Calories: 209
- Fat: 14.4g
- Carbohydrates: 11.4g
- Dietary Fiber: 1.8g
- Protein: 9.2g

Well-Done Moroccan Spiced Sweet Potatoes

Time: 19 minutes

Servings: 4

Ingredients:

- 1 pound of sweet potatoes, peeled and cut into 1-inch pieces
- 2 tablespoons of olive oil, coconut oil, or ghee
- ½ fresh lemon, juice
- 1 cup of water
- 1 tablespoons of ground organic coriander powder
- 1 tablespoon of ground organic cumin powder
- 1 tablespoon of chili powder
- 1 teaspoon of ground organic cinnamon powder
- 1 teaspoon of smoked paprika
- 1 teaspoon of ground ginger powder
- A small pinch of organic cayenne pepper powder
- 1 teaspoon of sea salt (to taste)
- 1 teaspoon of freshly ground black pepper (to taste)

Instructions:

- In a small bowl, add and mix all the spices and seasonings until well incorporated together.
- Add 1 cup of water and a steamer basket to your Instant Pot.
- Place the sweet potatoes on the steamer basket.
- Close and seal the lid on your Instant Pot. Press the "Manual" button and cook for 5 minutes on High Pressure.
- When the cooking is done, naturally release the pressure for 10 minutes and then quick release the remaining pressure. Transfer the sweet potatoes to a serving platter.
- Discard the water and remove the steamer basket from your Instant Pot.
- Press the "Sauté" function on your Instant Pot and add the olive oil or ghee.
- Once hot, working in batches if necessary, add the sweet potatoes and sauté until crispy.
- Sprinkle with the Moroccan spice mixture and drizzle with lemon juice.
- Repeat the process until all the sweet potatoes are perfectly cooked through.
- Serve and enjoy!

Nutrition information per serving:

- Calories: 196
- Fat: 7.2g
- Carbohydrates: 32.3g
- Dietary Fiber: 4.9g
- Protein: 1.8g

Pleasant Bacon-Wrapped Asparagus

Time: 16 minutes
Servings: 4
Ingredients:

- 1 pound of fresh thick Asparagus spears
- 8 bacon slices, cut in half
- 1 teaspoon of sea salt

Instructions:

- Add 2 cups of water and a steamer basket to your Instant Pot.
- Wrap the asparagus spears with bacon.
- Place the bacon-wrapped asparagus on top of the steamer basket.
- Close and seal the lid on your Instant Pot. Press the "Manual" button and cook for 3 minutes on High Pressure.
- When the cooking is done, quick release the pressure and remove the lid.
- Carefully remove the asparagus from your Instant Pot and transfer the bacon-wrapped asparagus to a serving platter. Sprinkle with salt.
- Serve and enjoy!

Nutrition information per serving:

- Calories: 228
- Fat: 16g
- Carbohydrates: 4.9g
- Dietary Fiber: 2.4g
- Protein: 16.6g

One of the Kind Mashed Garlic Sweet Potatoes

Time: 20 minutes
Servings: 8
Ingredients:

- 6 large sweet potatoes, peeled, washed, and cut into 1-inch chunks (You can leave the skin on if you like)
- 4 tablespoons of ghee or coconut butter
- 6 garlic cloves, minced
- 1 cup of homemade low-sodium organic chicken stock
- ½ cup of unsweetened coconut cream
- 1 teaspoon of dried thyme
- 1 teaspoon of dried oregano
- ½ teaspoon of ground organic cinnamon powder
- 1 teaspoon of sea salt (to taste)
- 1 teaspoon of freshly ground black pepper (to taste)

Instructions:

- Add the sweet potatoes, garlic, and water to your Instant Pot.
- Close and seal the lid on your Instant Pot. Press the "Manual" button and cook for 8 minutes on High Pressure.
- When the timer beeps, quick release the pressure and remove the lid.
- Stir in the coconut butter, unsweetened coconut cream, dried thyme, dried oregano, cinnamon powder, salt, and black pepper to your Instant Pot.
- Use a potato masher to mash the sweet potatoes until smooth and creamy.
- Serve and enjoy!

Nutrition information per serving:

- Calories: 187
- Fat: 7.9g
- Carbohydrates: 17.1g
- Dietary Fiber: 1.2g
- Protein: 6.3g

Wonderful Sautéed Swiss Chard with Nuts and Bacon

Time: 25 minutes
Servings: 6
Ingredients:

- 8 cups of fresh Swiss chard, roughly chopped
- ½ cup of organic homemade low-sodium chicken or vegetable stock
- 10 garlic cloves, crushed
- ½ cup of fresh raisins or dried cranberries
- ½ cup of pine nuts, unsalted
- 6 bacon slices, finely chopped
- 1 teaspoon of sea salt (to taste)
- 1 teaspoon of freshly ground black pepper (to taste)

Instructions:

- Press the "Sauté" function on your Instant Pot and add the bacon bits. Sauté until brown and crispy, stirring occasionally.
- Add the garlic and sauté for 1 minute, stirring occasionally.
- Turn off the "Sauté" function on your Instant Pot. Add the pine nuts, raisins, Swiss chard, and chicken stock to your Instant Pot.
- Close and seal the lid on your Instant Pot. Press the "Manual" button and cook for 1 minute on High Pressure.
- When the cooking is done, quick release the pressure and carefully remove the lid.
- Give a good stir and adjust the seasoning as needed.
- Serve and enjoy!

Nutrition information per serving:

- Calories: 201
- Fat: 16.3g
- Carbohydrates: 11.9g
- Dietary Fiber: 1g
- Protein: 6.3g

Crowd-Pleasing Buffalo Chicken Dip

Time: 1 hour
Servings: 8
Ingredients:

- 3 cups of raw cashews, soaked overnight
- 2 pounds of fresh boneless, skinless chicken thighs, breasts or tenderloins
- 1 (24-ounce) jar of Whole30-friendly chunky salsa
- 4 garlic cloves, minced
- 1 teaspoon of onion powder
- ¼ cup of homemade Whole30 friendly hot sauce
- 1 tablespoon of organic spicy brown mustard powder
- 1 teaspoon of smoked paprika
- 1 teaspoon of sea salt (to taste)
- 1 teaspoon of freshly ground black pepper (to taste)

Instructions:

- Add the chicken to the bottom of your Instant Pot. Pour the jar of chunky salsa over the chicken.
- Close and seal the lid on your Instant Pot. Press the "Manual" button and cook for 20 minutes on High Pressure.
- When the cooking is done, quick release the pressure and carefully remove the lid.
- Transfer the chicken to a serving platter and shred using two forks.
- In a food processor, add the garlic, cashews, onion powder, hot sauce, spicy brown mustard powder, smoked paprika, salt, and black pepper. Pulse until smooth.
- In a large bowl, add the shredded chicken and dip. Stir until well combined.
- Transfer the chicken-dip mixture to a greased baking dish.
- Bake in your oven until warm and crispy on the top.
- Serve and enjoy!

Nutrition information per serving:

- Calories: 490
- Fat: 27.4g
- Carbohydrates: 22.3g
- Dietary Fiber: 2.9g
- Protein: 42.1g

Mythical Sweet and Sour Cabbage

Time: 20 minutes
Servings: 4
Ingredients:

- 2 tablespoons of ghee, olive oil, or coconut oil
- 1 medium-sized red onion, finely chopped
- 4 garlic cloves, minced
- 1 medium-sized green cabbage, cored and shredded
- 1 medium-sized purple cabbage, cored and shredded
- 1 cup of unsweetened homemade fresh applesauce
- 1 tablespoon of apple cider vinegar
- 1 teaspoon of sea salt (to taste)
- 1 teaspoon of freshly ground black pepper (to taste)

Instructions:

- Press the "Sauté" function on your Instant Pot and add the ghee or oil.
- Once the display reads hot, add the red onion and sauté until translucent, stirring occasionally.
- Add the garlic and sauté for 1 minute or until fragrant, stirring occasionally.
- Add the green cabbage, purple cabbage, applesauce, apple cider vinegar, salt, and black pepper to your Instant Pot. Stir until well combined.
- Close and seal the lid on your Instant Pot. Press the "Manual" button on your Instant Pot and cook for 10 minutes on High Pressure.
- When the cooking is done, naturally release or quick release the pressure. Carefully remove the lid.
- Stir the cabbage again and adjust the seasoning as needed.
- Serve and enjoy!

Nutrition information per serving:

- Calories: 211
- Fat: 6.9g
- Carbohydrates: 36.8g
- Dietary Fiber: 12.7g
- Protein: 6.4g

Celebrated Stuffed Pepper Soup

Time: 23 minutes

Servings: 10

Ingredients:

- 1 pound of extra lean ground beef
- 2 sweet medium-sized red bell peppers, deseeded and finely chopped
- 2 sweet medium-sized green bell peppers, deseeded and finely chopped
- 2 cups of low sodium beef broth or water
- 1 (14-ounce) can of diced tomatoes, undrained
- 1 (6-ounce) can of tomato paste
- 1 (14-ounce) can of tomato sauce
- 1 cup of cauliflower florets, finely chopped
- 2 fresh bay leaves
- 3 medium-sized celery stalks, finely chopped
- 1 medium-sized yellow onion, finely chopped
- 4 garlic cloves, minced
- 1 tablespoon of organic smoked paprika or chili powder
- 1 teaspoon of Italian seasoning
- 1 teaspoon of dried thyme leaves
- 1 tablespoon of fresh parsley leaves, finely chopped
- 1 teaspoon of dried oregano leaves
- 2 teaspoons of sea salt (to taste)
- 1 teaspoon of freshly ground black pepper (to taste)

Instructions:

- Press the "Sauté" function on your Instant Pot.
- Once the cooking pot is hot, add the 1 pound of extra lean ground beef and the bay leaves to your Instant Pot. Cook for 4 minutes or until brown.
- Add the onion, garlic, celery, all the seasoning and spices to your Instant Pot. Sauté for 4 minutes, stirring frequently.
- Add the 4 bell peppers to your Instant Pot and give a good stir.
- Add the beef broth, diced tomatoes, tomato paste, tomato sauce, and finely chopped cauliflower florets to your Instant Pot.
- Place and seal the lid on your Instant Pot. Press the "Manual" button and cook for 4 minutes on High Pressure.
- When the cooking is done, naturally release the pressure for 15 minutes and then quick release the remaining pressure. Carefully remove the lid.
- Give the stuffed pepper soup a stir and adjust the seasoning as needed.
- Serve and enjoy!

Nutrition information per serving:

- Calories: 134
- Fat: 3.6g
- Carbohydrates: 9.6g
- Dietary Fiber: 2.4g
- Protein: 16.4g

Deliciously Acclaimed Broccoli and Sweet Potato Soup

Time: 23 minutes

Servings: 12

Ingredients:

- 5 pounds of sweet potatoes, peeled and chopped into medium-sized chunks
- ½ pound of bacon, finely chopped
- 4 cups of homemade low-sodium chicken broth or bone broth
- 3 cups of fresh broccoli florets
- 2 medium-sized fresh celery stalks, finely chopped
- 2 medium-sized carrots, finely chopped
- 3 tablespoons of avocado oil, coconut oil, or ghee
- 1 medium-sized yellow onions, finely chopped
- 3 garlic cloves, minced
- 2 cups of unsweetened coconut cream
- 1 teaspoon of sea salt (to taste)
- 1 teaspoon of freshly ground black pepper (to taste)

Instructions:

- Press the "Sauté" function on your Instant Pot and add the bacon bits. Cook until brown and crispy. Remove and set aside.
- Add the avocado oil, yellow onions, and garlic to your Instant Pot. Sauté until onions are lightly browned, stirring occasionally.
- Add the 5 pounds of sweet potato chunks, celery, carrots, 3 cups of broccoli florets, and 4 cups of chicken stock to your Instant Pot.
- Place and seal the lid on your Instant Pot. Press the "Manual" button and cook for 10 minutes on High Pressure.
- When the cooking is done, naturally release the pressure and remove the lid.
- Use a potato masher and mash the potatoes and broccoli until reached your desired consistency.
- Stir in the unsweetened coconut cream and adjust the seasoning as needed.
- Season with sea salt and ground black pepper. Stir in the cooked bacon bits.
- Serve and enjoy!

Nutrition information per serving:

- Calories: 451
- Fat: 18.8g
- Carbohydrates: 59.3g
- Dietary Fiber: 9.9g
- Protein: 13.3g

Gratifying Coconut Tomato Basil Soup

Time: 15 minutes
Servings: 8
Ingredients:

- 3 medium-sized celery ribs, finely chopped
- 3 medium-sized carrots, peeled and grated
- 1 medium-sized yellow onion, finely chopped
- 4 cups of homemade low-sodium chicken broth
- ½ cup of ghee
- ½ cup of almond flour or coconut flour
- 2 tablespoons of olive oil
- 2 cups of unsweetened coconut milk
- 1 cup of unsweetened shredded coconut flakes
- 1 (28-ounce) can of crushed tomatoes, undrained
- 1 (14.5-ounce) can of tomato sauce
- 1 tablespoon of dried basil
- 1 tablespoon of dried parsley
- 1 bay leaf
- 1 teaspoon of dried oregano
- 1 teaspoon of sea salt (to taste)
- 1 teaspoon of freshly ground black pepper (to taste)

Instructions:

- Press the "Sauté" function on your Instant Pot and add the olive oil.
- Once the display reads hot, add the onions and sauté for 2 minutes or until softened.
- Add the celery and carrots to your Instant Pot and sauté for an extra minute.
- Add the chicken broth and crushed tomatoes to your Instant Pot.
- Stir in the dried basil, dried parsley, bay leaf, dried oregano, sea salt, and freshly ground black pepper.
- Lock the lid and ensure the valve is sealed. Select the "Manual" setting and cook for 6 minutes on High Pressure.
- When the coking is done, naturally release the pressure for 10 minutes, then quick release any remaining pressure. Carefully remove the lid.
- Press the "Sauté" function on your Instant Pot and stir in the ghee and almond flour to the tomato mixture.
- Stir in the unsweetened coconut milk and unsweetened shredded coconut flakes to your Instant Pot until well combined.
- Allow to simmer for a couple of minutes until smooth and creamy. Adjust the seasoning as needed. Serve and enjoy!

Nutrition information per serving:

- Calories: 392
- Fat: 35.4g
- Carbohydrates: 15.9g
- Dietary Fiber: 6.8g
- Protein: 6.2g

Grandmother's Garden Chicken Soup

Time: 20 minutes
Servings: 8
Ingredients:

- 3 pounds of boneless, skinless fresh organic chicken breasts
- 2 tablespoons of olive oil
- 2 medium-sized yellow onions, finely chopped
- 2 medium-sized shallots, finely chopped
- 1 leek, thinly sliced
- 5 garlic cloves, minced
- 3 medium-sized carrots, peeled and chopped
- 3 medium-sized parsnips, peeled and chopped
- 8 cups of homemade low-sodium chicken stock
- 3 cups of kale, stemmed and chopped
- 1 tablespoon of fresh parsley, finely chopped
- 1 tablespoon of fresh dill, finely chopped
- 1 teaspoon of smoked paprika
- 1 teaspoon of sea salt (to taste)
- 1 teaspoon of freshly ground black pepper (to taste)

Instructions:

- Press the "Sauté" function on your Instant Pot and add the olive oil.
- Once the oil is hot, add the onions, shallots, leek, and garlic to your Instant Pot. Sauté for 5 minutes or until brown, stirring occasionally.
- Season the chicken with smoked paprika, salt, and black pepper and add to your Instant Pot.
- Add the carrots, parsnips, parsley, dill, and 8 cups of chicken stock to your Instant Pot.
- Lock the lid and ensure the valve is closed. Press the "Manual" button and cook for 12 minutes on High Pressure.
- When the cooking is done, naturally release the pressure and carefully remove the lid.
- Transfer the chicken to a serving platter and shred using two forks.
- Return the shredded chicken to your Instant Pot along with the kale.
- Place the lid on your Instant Pot and allow to sit for 5 minutes or until wilted.
- Serve and enjoy!

Nutrition information per serving:

- Calories: 365
- Fat: 9.4g
- Carbohydrates: 16.7g
- Dietary Fiber: 3.8g
- Protein: 51.9g

•

Full Body Cleansing Vegetable Soup

Time: 21 minutes
Servings: 4
Ingredients:

- 2 tablespoons of olive oil, coconut oil, or avocado oil
- 4 garlic cloves, minced
- 2 small-sized yellow onions, finely chopped
- 6 cups of low sodium vegetable stock or plain water
- 2 large carrots, peeled and chopped
- 2 medium-sized celery stalks, finely chopped
- 1 (14.5-ounce) can of crushed tomatoes, undrained
- 1 small fresh broccoli head, finely chopped
- 1 medium-sized fresh zucchini, chopped
- 1 medium-sized red pepper, chopped
- 1 medium-sized yellow pepper, chopped
- 2 teaspoons of Italian seasoning
- 1 teaspoon of sea salt (to taste)
- 1 teaspoon of freshly ground black pepper (to taste)

Instructions:

- Add all the ingredients to your Instant Pot besides the zucchini, bell pepper, and broccoli.
- Lock the lid and ensure the valve is closed.
- Press the "Manual" button and cook for 2 minutes on High Pressure.
- When the cooking is done, quick release the pressure and remove the lid.
- Stir the broccoli, zucchini, and bell pepper to your Instant Pot.
- Place the lid on your Instant Pot and allow to sit in your Instant Pot for 5 minutes or until the vegetables have softened.
- Serve and enjoy!

Nutrition information per serving:

- Calories: 223
- Fat: 0.8g
- Carbohydrates: 16.3g
- Dietary Fiber: 2.53g
- Protein: 13g

Heroic Creamy Cauliflower and Fennel Soup

Time: 30 minutes

Servings: 4

Ingredients:

- 1 pound of raw cauliflower florets, chopped
- 1 cup of unsweetened coconut milk
- 2 medium-sized fennel bulbs, stalks removed
- 1 tablespoon of coconut oil
- 3 garlic cloves, minced
- 1 medium-sized onion, finely chopped
- 3 cups of homemade low-sodium vegetable broth or bone broth
- 1 teaspoon of sea salt (to taste)
- 1 teaspoon of freshly ground black pepper (to taste)

Instructions:

- Press the "Sauté" function on your Instant Pot and add the coconut oil.
- Once the display reads hot, add the onion and sauté for 5 minutes or until translucent, stirring occasionally.
- Add the cauliflower, fennel, and garlic to your Instant Pot and sauté for 5 to 10 minutes or until golden brown, stirring occasionally.
- Add the vegetable broth and unsweetened coconut milk to your Instant Pot.
- Lock the lid and ensure the valve is closed. Press the "Manual" button and cook for 5 minutes on High Pressure.
- When the cooking is done, quick release the pressure and remove the lid.
- Use an immersion blender to blend the soup until smooth. Alternatively, you can transfer the contents to a blender and blend until reach your desired consistency.
- Season the soup with salt and black pepper.
- Serve and enjoy!

Nutrition information per serving:

- Calories: 276
- Fat: 19.1g
- Carbohydrates: 21.9g
- Dietary Fiber: 8.4g
- Protein: 9.2g

Well-Known Portuguese-Inspired Kale Soup

Time: 18 minutes
Servings: 8
Ingredients:

- 1 pound of ground turkey
- ½ pound of breakfast sausage, finely chopped
- 1 large bunch of fresh kale, stemmed and chopped
- 3 (14.5-ounce) can of diced tomatoes
- 6 cups of homemade low-sodium chicken stock
- 2 red bell pepper, deseeded and finely chopped
- 1 tablespoon of olive oil
- 1 large yellow onion, finely chopped
- 1 tablespoon of olive oil
- 2 garlic cloves, minced
- 3 large leeks, chopped
- 1 teaspoon of smoked paprika
- 1 tablespoon of dried oregano or parsley leaves
- 1 teaspoon of sea salt (to taste)
- 1 teaspoon of freshly ground black pepper (to taste)

Instructions:

- Press the "Sauté" function on your Instant Pot and add the olive oil.
- Once the display reads hot, add the leeks and onions to the cooking pot. Sauté for 3 to 5 minutes or until softened, stirring occasionally.
- Add the garlic and sauté for an extra minute, stirring occasionally.
- Add the ground turkey and finely chopped breakfast sausage. Sauté until brown, stirring occasionally. Turn off "Sauté" setting on your Instant Pot.
- Add the diced tomatoes, chicken stock, and red bell pepper to your Instant Pot.
- Lock the lid and ensure the valve is closed.
- Press the "Manual" button and cook for 6 minutes on High Pressure.
- When the cooking is done, naturally release the pressure and remove the lid.
- Stir in the chopped kale, smoked paprika, dried oregano, salt, and black pepper. Stir until the kale wilted.
- Serve and enjoy!

Nutrition information per serving:

- Calories: 254
- Fat: 12.9g
- Carbohydrates: 10.2g
- Dietary Fiber: 2.3g
- Protein: 24.4g

Celebrated Sweet Potato Soup

Time: 36 minutes

Servings: 6

Ingredients:

- 2 pounds of sweet potatoes, peeled and cut into 2-inch pieces
- 4 cups of low-sodium vegetable or chicken stock
- 2 cups of plain water
- 1 tablespoon of olive oil
- 1 medium-sized yellow onion, finely chopped
- 4 garlic cloves, minced
- 1 teaspoon of organic smoked paprika
- ½ teaspoon of organic ground cinnamon powder
- 1 teaspoon of sea salt (to taste)
- 1 teaspoon of freshly ground black pepper (to taste)
- ½ cup of unsweetened coconut cream

Instructions:

- Press the "Sauté" function on your Instant Pot and add 1 tablespoon of olive oil.
- Once the display reads hot, add the onions and sauté for 4 minutes or until translucent, stirring occasionally.
- Add the minced garlic and sauté for 1 minute, stirring occasionally.
- Add the 2 pounds of sweet potatoes, vegetable or chicken stock, smoked paprika, and cinnamon powder to your Instant Pot. Give a good stir.
- Place and seal the lid on your Instant Pot. Press the "Manual" button and cook for 10 minutes on High Pressure.
- When the cooking is done, quick release the pressure and carefully remove the lid.
- Use an immersion blender to blend the contents in your Instant Pot until smooth. Alternatively, you can transfer the contents to a blender or food processor and blend until reach your desired consistency.
- Stir in the unsweetened coconut milk, salt, and black pepper.
- Serve and enjoy!

Nutrition information per serving:

- Calories: 261
- Fat: 7.8g
- Carbohydrates: 46.1g
- Dietary Fiber: 7.1g
- Protein: 3.6g

Pleasurable and Healthy Green Chicken Soup

Time: 15 minutes

Servings: 8

Ingredients:

- 8 cups of homemade low-sodium chicken stock
- 1 pound of fresh boneless, skinless chicken breasts
- 1 large bunch of kale, stemmed and chopped
- 4 carrots, peeled and sliced
- 1 cup of shiitake mushrooms, sliced
- 1 tablespoon of dried oregano
- 1 teaspoon of onion powder
- 1 teaspoon of garlic powder
- 1 teaspoon of sea salt (to taste)
- 1 teaspoon of freshly ground black pepper (to taste)

Instructions:

- In a blender or food processor, add 6 cups of homemade low-sodium chicken stock and a large bunch of chopped kale. Pulse until smooth and relatively creamy.
- Add the kale mixture and the remaining ingredients to your Instant Pot.
- Place and seal the lid on your Instant Pot. Press the "Manual" button and cook for 8 minutes on High Pressure.
- When the cooking is done, naturally release the pressure and remove the lid.
- Transfer the chicken to a serving platter and shred using two forks.
- Return the shredded chicken to your Instant Pot and stir until well combined with the kale-stock mixture.
- Serve and enjoy

Nutrition information per serving:

- Calories: 126
- Fat: 2.3g
- Carbohydrates: 7.5g
- Dietary Fiber: 1.3g
- Protein: 18.6g

Lovely Polish-Inspired Cabbage Soup

Time: 21 minutes

Servings: 6

Ingredients:

- 1 large head of fresh green cabbage, cored and thinly sliced
- 2 pounds of sauerkraut, rinsed
- 1 pound of pork, sliced into ¼-inch strips
- 2 tablespoons of olive oil
- 1 (14-ounce) can of diced tomatoes, undrained
- 1 (14-ounce) can of tomato sauce
- 4 cups of low-sodium chicken stock or vegetable stock
- 1 teaspoon of onion powder
- 1 teaspoon of garlic powder
- 1 teaspoon of sea salt (to taste)
- 1 teaspoon of freshly ground black pepper (to taste)

Instructions:

- Press the "Sauté" function on your Instant Pot and add the olive oil.
- Once the display reads hot, working in batches if necessary, add the pork strips and sauté until brown. Turn off "Sauté" function and add all the pork strips back to the inner pot.
- Add the sauerkraut, green cabbage, diced tomatoes, tomato sauce, chicken stock, onion powder, and garlic powder to your Instant Pot.
- Lock the lid and ensure the valve is closed on your Instant Pot. Press the "Manual" button and cook for 15 minutes on High Pressure.
- When the cooking is done, naturally release the pressure and carefully remove the lid.
- Give the cabbage soup a good stir and season the soup with salt and pepper.
- Serve and enjoy!

Nutrition information per serving:

- Calories: 245
- Fat: 8.3g
- Carbohydrates: 20.9g
- Dietary Fiber: 9.8g
- Protein: 24.7g

Chapter 10: Amazing Desserts and Sweets Recipes

Magnificent Coconut Custard

Time: 35 minutes

Servings: 4

Ingredients:

- 4 large eggs
- ¾ cup of unsweetened coconut milk
- ½ cup of unsweetened organic coconut cream
- A pinch of salt to bring out the flavor
- 1/3 cup of swerve
- ½ teaspoon of organic ground cinnamon

Instructions:

- In a large bowl, add the 4 large eggs, unsweetened coconut milk, unsweetened coconut cream, a pinch of salt, swerve, and cinnamon. Stir using a spatula or spoon until well blended together.
- In a heat-safe dish or 4 soufflé dishes, pour the blended coconut mixture and tightly cover with aluminum foil to prevent liquid from settling on the top.
- Pour 2 cups of water and add a trivet to the Instant Pot.
- Place the heat-proof dish or soufflé dishes on top of the trivet.
- Place and seal the lid on the Instant. Manually set the cooking time for 30 minutes on High Pressure.
- When the cooking is finished, allow a full natural release before removing the lid.
- Remove the heat-proof dish or soufflé dishes from the Instant Pot and refrigerate until completely cool and the coconut custard is set.
- Serve and enjoy!

Nutrition information per serving:

- Calories: 234
- Fat: 22.6g
- Carbohydrates: 14.7g
- Dietary Fiber: 1.86g
- Protein: 8.1g

Effortless Banana Custard

Time: 37 minutes

Servings: 5

Ingredients:

- ½ cup of unsweetened coconut cream
- 2 large bananas, mashed
- 3 large eggs
- 1 cup of fresh large banana slices (for topping)
- ½ teaspoon of organic ground cinnamon
- A pinch of salt to bring out the flavor
- 1 cup of unsweetened coconut milk

Instructions:

- In a large bowl, add the 3 large eggs, mashed bananas, unsweetened coconut cream, unsweetened coconut milk, ground cinnamon, and a pinch of salt. Stir until well blended together. Alternatively, you can add the ingredients to a blender and blend until smooth.
- In 5 heat-safe ramekins, divide the banana mixture among the 5 ramekins.
- Pour 2 cup of water and a trivet inside your Instant Pot.
- Place all 6 ramekins on top of the ramekin and cover with aluminum foil.
- Place and seal the lid on the Instant Pot. Manually set the cooking time to 28 minutes on High Pressure.
- When the cooking is done, allow a natural release for 10 minutes and then manually release the remaining pressure. Remove the lid and carefully set the ramekins aside.
- Refrigerate the banana custards until completely cool. Top with fresh banana slices.
- Serve and enjoy!

Nutrition information per serving:

- Calories: 228
- Fat: 17.3g
- Carbohydrates: 20.1g
- Dietary Fiber: 3.3g
- Protein: 2.4g

Overqualified Berry Jam

Time: 20 minutes
Servings: 14
Ingredients:

- 1 cup of blueberries, washed
- 1 apple, cored, peeled, and chopped
- 1 pound of fresh strawberries, washed, trimmed and cut in half
- ¼ cup of freshly squeezed orange juice
- 2 tablespoons of water
- A pinch of salt to bring out the flavor

Instructions:

- Add 1 pound of strawberries, 1 cup of blueberries, 1 apple, freshly squeezed orange juice, water and pinch of salt to your Instant Pot.
- Close and seal the lid in your Instant Pot. Press the "Manual" button on your Instant Pot and set the time to 1 minute on High Pressure.
- When the cooking is done, allow a full natural release for 10 minutes then quick release any remaining pressure. Carefully remove the lid.
- Use a potato masher to mash the berry mixture until reached your desired consistency.
- Press the "Sauté" function on your Instant Pot and allow to simmer until thickened, stirring regularly with a wooden spoon.
- Turn off "Sauté" function and allow the berry jam to cool inside your refrigerator.
- Serve and enjoy!

Nutrition information per serving:

- Calories: 27
- Fat: 0.2g
- Carbohydrates: 6.7g
- Dietary Fiber: 1.3g
- Protein: 0.4g

Beautiful Cinnamon Apple Slices

Time: 40 minutes
Servings: 8
Ingredients:

- 3 pounds of apples, washed, peeled, cored, and sliced
- 2 teaspoons of organic ground cinnamon
- 2 tablespoons of cashew butter, coconut butter, almond butter, or ghee
- 3 tablespoons of water

Instructions:

- Add all the apple slices, ground cinnamon, 3 tablespoons of water, and nut butter to your Instant Pot. Stir until well combined.
- Place and seal the lid on your Instant Pot. Press the "Manual" button and set the time to 2 minutes on High Pressure.
- When the cooking is done, quick release the pressure and remove the lid.
- Serve and enjoy!

Nutrition information per serving:

- Calories: 47
- Fat: 0.3g
- Carbohydrates: 10.8g
- Dietary Fiber: 1.9g
- Protein: 0.4g

Everyday Sautéed Peaches and Apples

Time: 20 minutes
Servings: 4
Ingredients:

- 4 large ripe peaches, pitted and cut into 8 wedges
- 4 large apples, washed, cored, and cut into 8 wedges
- 4 tablespoons of almond butter, cashew butter, coconut butter, or ghee
- 1 tablespoon of organic ground cinnamon
- A pinch of salt to bring out the flavor

Instructions:

- Press the "Sauté" button on your Instant Pot and add the nut butter.
- Once the butter has melted, add the peaches and apples. Cook until the fruit is warmed through, stirring occasionally.
- Add the ground cinnamon and pinch of salt to the peaches and apples. Stir until well coated together.
- Continue to cook the peaches and apples until softened, about 3 to 5 minutes.
- Serve and enjoy!

Nutrition information per serving:

- Calories: 273
- Fat: 9.9g
- Carbohydrates: 47.9g
- Dietary Fiber: 9.5g
- Protein: 37.8g

Victorious Chocolate Cupcakes

Time: 20 minutes
Servings: 6
Ingredients:

- 2 large ripe bananas, peeled
- 1 large apple, peeled, cored and chopped
- 1 cup of almond butter or any other alternatives
- 2 large eggs
- 6 pitted dates
- ¼ cup of unsweetened organic cocoa powder
- 1 teaspoon of baking soda
- 1 teaspoon of organic ground cinnamon
- A pinch of salt to bring out to flavor

Instructions:

- In a blender, add the bananas, apple, almond butter, eggs, pitted dates, unsweetened cocoa powder, baking soda, ground cinnamon, and a pinch of salt to a blender or food processor. Blend until smooth.
- Grease 6 ramekins with nonstick cooking spray and divide the batter among the 6 ramekins.
- Add 2 cups of water and a trivet to your Instant Pot.
- Place the ramekins on top of the trivet and cover with aluminum foil.
- Place and seal the lid on your Instant Pot. Press the "Manual" button and set the time to 15 minutes on High Pressure.
- When the cooking is done, naturally release the pressure and carefully remove the lid.
- Carefully remove the ramekins and allow to cool.
- Serve and enjoy!

Nutrition information per serving:

- Calories: 126
- Fat: 3.9g
- Carbohydrates: 22.9g
- Dietary Fiber: 3.9g
- Protein: 4.1g

Fabulous Berry Compote

Time: 20 minutes
Servings: 4
Ingredients:

- 1 pound of fresh blueberries, raspberries or blackberries, washed
- 1 pound of fresh strawberries, washed, trimmed and cut in half
- 1 teaspoon of organic ground nutmeg
- 1 teaspoon of organic ground cinnamon
- 2 teaspoons of fresh orange juice
- 2 teaspoons of fresh lemon juice

Instructions:

- Add the fresh berries and strawberries to your Instant Pot. Stir until well combined.
- Stir in the whole nutmeg, ground cinnamon, orange juice, and lemon juice to your Instant Pot. Give a good stir.
- Place and seal the lid on your Instant Pot. Press the "Manual" button on your Instant Pot and set the time to 1 minutes.
- When the cooking is done, allow for a natural release method for 15 minutes and carefully remove the lid.
- Allow the berry compote to thicken until cool.
- Serve and enjoy!

Nutrition information per serving:

- Calories: 103
- Fat: 0.8g
- Carbohydrates: 25.3g
- Dietary Fiber: 5.3g
- Protein: 1.7g

Nicest Homemade Caramel-Applesauce

Time: 22 minutes
Servings: 8
Ingredients:

- 3 pounds of apples, peeled, cored and sliced
- 3 tablespoons of ghee
- 1 cup of water
- ½ teaspoon of salt
- 1 tablespoon of fresh lemon or lime juice
- 1 teaspoon of organic ground cinnamon (more as needed)

Instructions:

- Add the sliced apples, water, salt, lemon juice, ground cinnamon, and ghee to your Instant Pot. Give a good a stir.
- Place and seal the lid on your Instant Pot. Press the "Manual" button and set the time to 8 minutes on High Pressure.
- When the cooking is done, quick release the pressure and carefully remove the lid.
- Use a potato masher to mash the apple mixture until reached your desired consistency.
- Stir in more ground cinnamon as needed.
- Serve and enjoy!

Nutrition information per serving:

- Calories: 86
- Fat: 4g
- Carbohydrates: 14.3g
- Dietary Fiber: 2.1g
- Protein: 3.3g

Perfect Banana Foster

Time: 10 minutes
Servings: 4
Ingredients:

- 4 large bananas, peeled and cut into slices
- 1 cup of pineapples, chopped
- ½ cup of almond butter, coconut butter, cashew butter, or ghee
- ¼ cup of water
- ¼ cup of pineapple juice
- A pinch of salt
- 1 ½ teaspoons of organic ground cinnamon

Instructions:

- Stir the water and pineapple juice into your Instant Pot.
- Add the nut butter, pinch of salt and cinnamon. Give a good stir.
- Stir the sliced bananas and chopped pineapples to your Instant Pot.
- Sprinkle the ground cinnamon over the banana and pineapple pieces.
- Place and seal the lid on your Instant Pot. Press the "Manual" button and set the time to 8 minutes on High Pressure.
- When the cooking is done, manually release the pressure and remove the lid.
- Transfer the contents to a serving bowl and allow to cool.
- Serve and enjoy!

Nutrition information per serving:

- Calories: 148
- Fat: 1.7g
- Carbohydrates: 34.8g
- Dietary Fiber: 3.9g
- Protein: 2g

Favorite Smooth Pumpkin Custard

Time: 23 minutes

Servings: 6

Ingredients:

- 1 (15-ounce) can of pumpkin puree
- 1 ¾ cups of unsweetened coconut milk
- 4 large eggs
- 2 tablespoons of almond butter, coconut butter, almond butter, or ghee
- A pinch of salt to bring out the flavor
- 1 teaspoon of ground organic cinnamon
- ¼ cup of sliced almonds
- ¼ cup of chopped walnuts or pecans
- 2 large fresh bananas

Instructions:

- In a large bowl, add the pumpkin puree, unsweetened coconut milk, non-dairy butter, 4 large eggs, ground cinnamon, and a pinch of salt. Stir with a wooden spoon until well blended together. Alternatively, you can add the ingredients to a food processor and pulse until completely smooth.
- Add 1 cup of water and a trivet to your Instant Pot.
- In 6 heat-safe ramekins or soufflé dishes, divide and add the pumpkin mixture among the 6 dishes.
- Place the 6 dishes on top of the trivet and cover with aluminum foil.
- Place and seal the lid on your Instant Pot. Press the "Manual" button and set the time to 13 minutes on High Pressure.
- When the cooking is done, allow to naturally release the pressure for 10 minutes then quick release the remaining pressure. Remove the lid and carefully set the dishes aside.
- Refrigerate the pumpkin custard until cool or you can serve warm.
- Enjoy!

Nutrition information per serving:

- Calories: 139.6
- Fat: 2.6g
- Carbohydrates: 28.12g
- Dietary Fiber: 2.3g
- Protein: 3.4g

Conclusion

Thank you again for reading my book, "30 Day Whole Food Challenge".

After reading this book, you finally got to realize what the Whole30 diet is, how you can get started, how to stick with it, and 100 Whole30 recipes using your Instant Pot. You also have in possession a 30-day meal plan and tips for succeeding in the Whole30. With this said, I am sure that you will meet your health goals using this book.

Finally, if you enjoyed this book or find something of value from it, please take the time to leave an honest review on Amazon. Recommend to your friends and family. This all would be greatly appreciated.

Thank you, and the best of luck on your Whole30 diet journey!